Mad·House

The Hidden History of Insane Asylums In 19th Century New York

MICHAEL T. KEENE

WM

Published by Willow Manor Publishing

Fredericksburg, V.A. 22406

www.willowmanorpublishing.com

First published 2013

Manufactured in the United States

LCCN 2013932682

Library of Congress Catalogue-in-Publication Data

Keene, Michael.

Mad House: The Hidden History of Insane Asylums
In 19th Century New York

Michael Keene

p.cm.

Includes bibliographical references.

ISBN 978-1-939688-01-9

1.History—New York (state). 2. Psychiatric Hospitals—New York (state). 3. Mental Illness—New York (state). 4. 19th Century—New York (state). 5. Asylums—New York (state).

Anecdotes. I. Title

Contents

To my wife

"Still mad about you."

Mad Hatter said to Alice: "Why is a raven like a writing-desk?"

"I give it up," Alice replied: "What's the answer?"

"I haven't the slightest idea" said the Hatter

Lewis Carroll, Alice-In-Wonderland

Introduction

Earlier this year I took my grandson to a Boy Scout camping trip at Camp Babcock-Hovey in Ovid, New York, located about 45 miles south east of Rochester. As we were entering town I spotted a sign that read, 'Willard Drug Treatment Center'. Something about the name 'Willard' sent a chill down my spine. At the time I didn't know why but the feeling stayed with me for the rest of the ride back...Willard? Willard? Where had I heard that name before?

When I finally arrived home, I went directly to my computer and began to Google "Willard". After a few minutes I found it, "Willard Drug Treatment Center", was a facility for the treatment of drug-addicted prisoners. But prior to becoming a drug treatment center, Willard had been a psychiatric hospital, and back in the 19th-century it was known as, "Willard Asylum for the Insane". But the history of 'Willard' involved more than just being a hospital that treated the 'insane'. It was also considered one of the most infamous psychiatric hospitals in New York State. The reasons for this are many (see chapter 11) but when the original Willard psychiatric hospital finally shuttered its doors in 1995, approximately 5700 bodies were found in unmarked graves, buried near the facility. All were former Willard patients!

As I grappled with the enormity of this revelation, I not only began to delve deeper into the history of 'Willard', but into the history of 19th-century New York 'insane asylums' in general. Frankly, not only did I find the material fascinating, but the subject also seemed like a great topic and natural 'fit' for my next book as I had previously written about true crime mysteries centered in New York during the 19th century. What better subject to write about than the most profound mystery of all; the mystery of the mind?

As I thought more about the project of writing a book about the history of insane asylums, I began to reflect on my own personal experiences in the psychiatric field. For several years I was employed initially as a psychiatric social worker and then later as the director of an outpatient mental health clinic. My first position in the early 1970's was with one of the first community mental health centers ever established in New York, (Arden Hill Mental Health Center in Goshen, New York). Then in the late 1970's I became the director of two outpatient mental health clinics in rural southern Georgia. Coincidentally, this also was a point in time that New York was beginning to transition from large state hospitals and long-term inpatient care for treating the mentally ill, to community based mental health centers and their emphasis on short-term crisis intervention.

I then also began to contemplate my own family history of mental illness. Like most people, I suspect, I had a close relative who had endured severe psychiatric problems during the 1960's. At a fairly young age, I was to become aware of such psychiatric symptoms and diagnoses as schizophrenia, hallucinations and psychosis, and psychiatric 'care' consisting of involuntary commitment, electro-shock therapy, and lobotomy.

As I continued to delve further into the history of the treatment of mental illness, the more I began to appreciate that society, and New York in particular, had in a way come 'full circle on the issue'. Until the ratification of the 1828 County Poorhouse Act, which was the first attempt at providing basic humanitarian services for the poor and the insane, life for the mentally ill was generally one of abuse, neglect and sometimes even torture. But county poorhouses, even with their best of intentions, would soon become 'dumping grounds' for people whose problems ranged from the indigent, the orphaned, the infirmed, 'the mental deficient', and the insane. It wasn't until the mid nineteenth-century and the establishment of large state asylums with their emphasis on 'moral therapy' that the care of the mentally ill began to slowly improve. But the large asylums very success's carried the seeds of their own demise as overcrowding and shortages, both of money and material, caused the system to become unwieldy and self defeating. A half a

Introduction

century later, beginning in the 1950's, there was a shift back to the concept of community based care with the advent of the Community Mental Health Center Act and the concept of, 'milieu therapy'.

As I explored the historical context of 'insane asylums', I began to discover not only an intriguing period in New York history but an extraordinary array of characters. They included not only the visionaries and reformers who were at the forefront of the state asylum system and the resulting initial improvements in mental health care, but also the patients who became the 'beneficiaries' of these changes and whose humanity opens a window to a unique perspective in the telling of this story.

It was during this time of asylum building, that we witnessed folly, sometimes mistreatment, and dare I say, even madness, in the care of the mentally ill. But it was also a time that promised hope and healing. It was the time of the Mad House, and the Hidden History of the Insane Asylums in 19th Century New York.

Chapter 1

Architecture of Madness

The discovery of trephine skulls in archaeological sites has proven there were attempts to treat mental illness as far back as 5000 BCE. Trephining, or trepanning, was evidenced as early as Neolithic times when a hole, or trephine, was chipped into the skull of the patient with crude stone or rock axe-shaped instruments. The general belief was that evil spirits had invaded the patient's skull (and therefore his life, his thoughts, and his behaviors) and would be automatically eliminated through the exit hole and he then would be cured. Some patients survived for many years as attested to by the discovery of skulls with healed openings. This procedure evolved through the years as an acceptable method of treating skull fractures, migraines, and mental illness. Ancient doctors served as

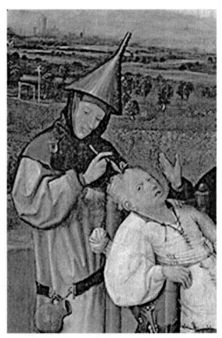

Evidence of Trephining found as early as prehistoric times. It was believed the practice would cure epileptic seizures, migraines and mental disorders

priests as well, and in Mesopotamia, the mentally ill were treated with pseudo-magic rituals to remove traces of demonic possession, which many believed accompanied mental aberrations. Exorcisms, incantations, atonement, prayers and other rituals were utilized to force evil spirits out. Bribery, threats, punishment, and food deprivation, were also attempted to help rid the patient of the presence of evil. (1)

The Hebrews believed God punished humans by inflicting illness upon them because of their sins against God, whose wrath could literally cause diseases. At the same time, God was credited with being the supreme healer and some special Hebrew priests had specific methods of appealing to their Higher Power for cures. The Persians were convinced demons caused all illnesses and they believed good deeds and pure thoughts could protect humans from sickness and disease. (2)

Ancient Egyptians

The most logical-thinking of the ancient civilizations in regards to mental illness were the Egyptians who suggested recreational activities such as dance,

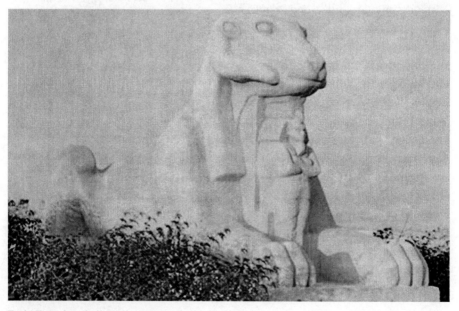

Early Egyptians believed recreational activities would reduce symptoms. Would later become the basis of homeopathy medicine.

painting, concerts, etc., might help relieve symptoms and keep the patient's concentration more closely focused on normalcy. They were also advanced in the fields of surgery, medicine, and the workings of the different parts of the human body. Two ancient papyri dating back to the 16th century BCE clearly document the treatment of wounds with surgery and identified the human brain as the site of cognitive functions. (3)

Hippocrates

Hippocrates was a brilliant Greek physician who denied the popular belief that mental illness was caused by supernatural forces. He presented the idea of natural occurrences in the human body as the cause, specifically pathology in the brain. Hippocrates and later, Galen, a Roman physician, introduced the idea of four essential fluids in the human body - blood, phlegm, bile, and black bile - when combined in different amounts, produced the differing personalities of all individuals. Therefore, through the middle Ages, an imbalance of these four liquids was believed to cause different mental illnesses. In order to correct this imbalance, patients were given emetics, were bled using leeches, given laxatives, or special purges to induce vomiting. Other treatments extracted blood from the forehead, or pulled "corrupted" humors away from the brain by tapping the cephalic veins. Customized diets were often recommended as well, such as "cooling and diluting" diets consisting of salad greens, barley water, milk , and avoiding wine and red meat. (4)

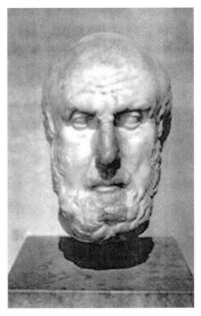

Hippocrates (460 BC-377 BC) Ancient Greek physician who believed that demons were not the cause of insanity but it was a medical condition requiring treatment.

Architecture of Madness

The First Asylums

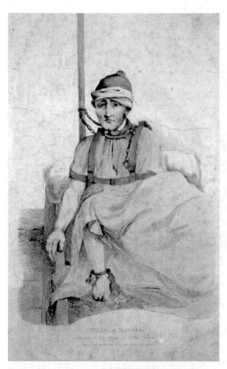

Forced restraint was invented by the French in 1790. Eventually led to the development of the 'holding chair' and the 'straight jacket'.

Custody and care of the mentally ill was typically left to the patient's family, but occasionally outside intervention occurred. In 792 Baghdad, the first mental hospital was officially established. Later, others were founded in Aleppo and Damascus. The insane who were in the custody of family members would often suffer abuse. Many families hid the mentally ill in cellars, or barns and others were abandoned and left to survive as beggars and vagrants. (5)

The social stigma attached to the mentally ill was more pronounced in countries that put extreme emphasis on family honor and relied on marriages to form alliances. In China, the mentally ill were thought to indicate there was an evil behavior being enacted by the family behind closed doors, so they were concealed by their families, forever if possible. Some communities believed the mental illness might be contagious. In Greece, for example, even now a mentally ill family member indicates a possible flawed bloodline and is a threat to the family's status as an honorable unit. Many of the insane were regarded as dangerous and were imprisoned, often for life. During the Middle Ages in Europe punishment was used to "rid bodies" of the evils of insanity and others were flogged and chased out of town. But also during this time there were humanistic physicians, medical astrologers, apothecaries and traditional healers to help the mentally ill. Prayers, charms, amulets and other mystical treatments were used as well. Sedatives during the 17th century such as opium grains, unguents, and laudanum were believed to dull the torment of mental illness. (6)

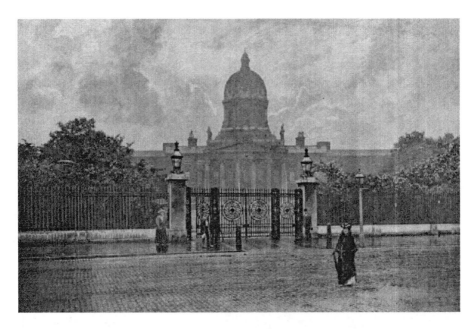

Bethlem Royal Hospital. England's oldest psychiatric institution founded in 1247. Would remain an active hospital for 600 years. The word 'bedlam' is derived from its name.

The Royal Hospital of Bethlehem

London's Bethlem Royal Hospital, long called Bedlam, is believed to be one of the oldest mental institutions in the world. It was founded by Christians in 1247 to shelter and care for homeless people, but gradually began to focus on those considered 'mad'. Patients did not often stay longer than 12 months. Ex-patients were called 'Bedlamites' and were licensed to beg on main routes between towns. Bedlam came under the control of the City of London in 1547. It was the only public mental institution in England until well into the 1800s.

Despite its large reputation, Bedlam remained small for centuries - there were no more than 24 patients in 1620. Its location near the walls of London (on land now occupied by Liverpool Street Station) and status as a public institution ensured a stream of visitors eager to view 'madness'. In 1676 Bedlam moved to a new and larger building at Moorfields with a baroque facade by natural philosopher Robert Hooke that was designed to impress visitors. Commentators have noted visitors and artists often projected onto Bedlam their hopes and fears about 'madness'.

Bedlam's high profile saw it repeatedly criticized and mired in scandal. Some of its most outspoken patients were confined because their political enemies wanted to silence or discredit them. Government inquiries into the abuse of Bedlam patients inspired reforms up through the 1800s. 'Bedlam' came to describe any out-of-control situation.

The hospital moved again in 1815 to improve patient conditions. It was further away from the city centre, so patients had more space for indoor and outdoor activities. This was central to the concept of 'moral treatment', a true revolution in the field of mental health care. In 1930, Bedlam moved to its current home, a large campus in the London suburbs which houses patients in small, separate, home-like buildings rather than a single fortress-like structure. Bethlem Royal Hospital is now a research and treatment centre, and its small museum holds a renowned collection of art made by people diagnosed with mental illness.(7)

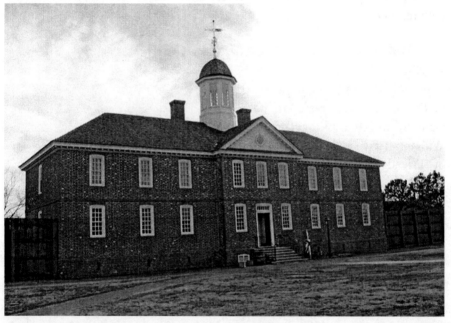

Eastern State Hospital founded in Williamsburg, Virginia in 1773. It would become the first insane asylum in the United States.

Philippe Pinel

Other countries soon began to establish asylums for the insane such as in Mexico where San Hippolito was built in 1566 - claiming the title of the first asylum in the Americas. In a suburb of Paris, La Madison de Chareton was the first mental facility in France. In 1784, the Lunatics' Tower in Vienna, became a showplace. The staff lived in opulent rooms in the elaborately decorated round tower and patients were housed in the spaces between the walls and as at Bedlam, were put on display for the public's amusement.

Philippe Pinel introduced one of the most significant reforms to occur in the mental health field. During the year 1792, Pinel took charge of the asylum La Bicetre to prove mentally ill patients would show better and faster improvement if they were treated with kindness and consideration. Noise, filth, and abuse were eliminated and patients were unchained, provided with ample living spaces, allowed to exercise freely on the grounds and regarded with respect. (8)

The York Retreat

The Retreat at York led the world in the humane treatment of the mentally ill. It was founded by William Tuke and the Society of Friends (Quakers) in 1792, and opened in 1796. Tuke was inspired by seeing the appalling conditions in York Lunatic Asylum when a Quaker from Leeds, Hannah Mills, died there.

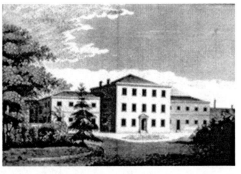

York Retreat founded in 1796 by William Tuke. Originally an institution for Quakers became a model for the moral treatment of the mentally ill.

Ill treatment of patients was widely accepted in the asylums of the time. Many believed that 'lunatics' were insensitive to hot and cold, almost sub-human, like animals. Beatings and confinement were accepted practice, as was underfeeding patients. In 1786, Joseph Townsend wrote on the subject, "Hunger will tame the fiercest animals, it will teach decency and civility, obedience and subjection to the most perverse".

It was in response to these attitudes that the Retreat was born, based instead on the Quaker principles of self-control, compassion and respect. Originally, the institution was primarily for Quakers to be treated in an environment sympathetic to their needs. However, it did open its doors to non-Quakers, although they were charged a higher weekly residence fee.

The Retreat marks the beginning of the move away from chains and fetters to gentler restraint such as the straight jacket. The Quakers did not see the insane as animals, but believed the 'inner light of God' to be present in all. The patients were not to be beaten or chained up, but were considered as children and the Retreat as a loving family environment to bring patients back to reason, and recovery.

Another innovation was 'The Appendage', a half-way house 'for those needing least supervision'.

This radical approach began a series of reforms and greater understanding in mental health and psychiatry in the nineteenth century. Textbooks today still refer to the Retreat. Julia Unwin of the Joseph Rowntree Foundation said, "It is perhaps easy for us looking back from our apparently enlightened times not to recognize the true impact of this extraordinary leap forward in the care of mentally ill people and the bravery of Tuke in pioneering it."(9)

Moral Treatment

With a humanitarian system firmly entrenched in the work of Pinel and Tuke, moral management eventually was introduced in America as a "wide-ranging method of treatment focusing on a patient's social, individual, and occupational needs." When applied to asylum care, the concept of moral therapy concentrated on the mentally ill individual's spiritual and moral development, as well as the rehabilitation of their character. This was achieved by encouraging patients to engage in manual labor, physical activity and spiritual awareness.

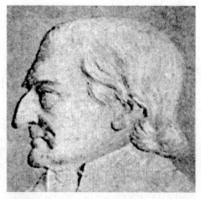

William Tuke (1732-1822) was a English businessman, philanthropist, and Quaker. He was instrumental in the development of more humane treating people with mental disorders.

Moral therapy worked well as far as it went but it failed to remain viable as the growth and sheer size of asylums escalated. Some institutions would begin with only thirty or forty patients and then rapidly grow to hundreds, and by the latter part of the 19th-century, sometimes thousands. This led to an overextension of resources, both in terms of supplies and staff, and then neglect and abuse would ensue. (10)

Dorothea Dix

There are few cases in history where a social movement can be attributed to the work of a single individual. Dorothea Dix, arguably, was such that person. She was a teacher and social reformer who worked tirelessly for the betterment for treatment of the mentally ill. Her life goals were not well defined; she simply did whatever would best help people. By the time she was thirty-nine, she had traveled to over half of the states in the country and most of Europe inspecting 'insane asylums' for evidence of mistreatment. The changes she helped usher-in fundamentally improved the lives of the mentally ill and are still felt today.

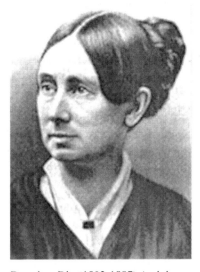

Dorothea Dix (1802-1887) Activist on behalf of the indigent insane, helped create the first generation of American mental asylums. During the Civil War, she served as Superintendent of Army Nurses.

Dorothea Lynde Dix was born on April 4, 1802 in the town of Hampden, Maine. She was the first child of three born to Joseph Dix and Mary Bigelow Dix. Her father was an itinerant Methodist preacher. Her family life can only be described as abusive and violent. Her mother was not in good mental health and her father was an alcoholic. Once the Dix family settled in Worcester they had two more children, Joseph and Charles. Almost immediately Dorothea began to care for her smaller brothers. Later in life she commented that "I never knew childhood."

Architecture of Madness

Social Reformer

After an early career as a teacher, Dorothea's concerns for the indigent and the mentally ill would begin when she entered the East Cambridge Jail, where she had volunteered to teach a Sunday school class for women inmates. Upon entering the jail she witnessed images that changed her life forever. Within the confines of the jail she observed prostitutes, drunks, criminals, the 'retarded' and the mentally ill, housed together in unheated, unfurnished, and foul-smelling quarters. When asked why the jail was in this condition she was told, "The insane do not feel heat or cold".

Dorothea's views about the treatment of the mentally ill were radical for her time. The popular belief was that the insane could never be cured and living in dreadful conditions was good enough. However, Dix attempted to show that mental illness wasn't incurable. Dix stated that "some may say these things cannot be remedied, these furious maniacs are not to be raised from these base conditions. I know they are...I could give many examples. One such is a young woman who was for years 'a raging maniac' chained in a cage and whipped to control her acts and words. She was helped by a husband and wife who agreed to take care of her in their home and slowly she recovered her senses." Although Dorothea didn't know the mental processes that were occurring within these individuals she knew that improving their conditions would help.

Dix would soon travel to other states and proceeded to visit and investigate other jails and almshouses. Although her health was very poor, she managed to cover every state on the east side of the Mississippi River. In all she played a major role in the founding of 32 mental hospitals, 15 schools for the feeble minded, a school for the blind, and numerous training facilities for nurses. Her efforts were an indirect inspiration for the building of many additional institutions for the mentally ill. She was also instrumental in establishing libraries in prisons and other social welfare institutions.

In 1881 the state hospital in Trenton, New Jersey, opened. This was the first hospital that was initiated and built through her efforts. Since her health was failing she admitted herself into the hospital. However, with her decline, she remained in the hospital for six years. Her death on July 17, 1887 ended a career that was unique in its singleness of purpose and magnitude of accomplishment.

Dorothea Dix has been described as the most effective advocate of humanitarian reform in American mental institutions during the nineteenth century. However, her achievements are only mentioned in five of the current fifty-three textbooks covering the history of psychology. The reason given for this is that she did not contribute to our understanding of the nature of mental disorders. Though this may seem something hard to fathom Dorothea Dix herself probably would have wanted it this way. She was inconspicuous with her work, and did not place her name on most of her publications. She refused to have hospitals named after her. She felt expressions of praise and gratitude for her work caused her embarrassment. In later years, during her retirement, she refused to talk about her achievements, wanting them to "rest in silence". (11)

In part, due to the work of Dorothea Dix and her view of more humane treatment, a radical change in public attitudes towards mental illness began to take place, specifically as to 'where' patients should be treated. And it is the 'where', and the creation of large asylums that housed and treated the insane for almost a hundred years that will now become the focus of this story. The individual most responsible for the phenomena of asylum building was Dr. Thomas Story Kirkbride. (12)

Dr. Thomas Story Kirkbride

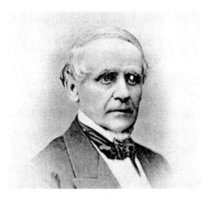

Thomas Story Kirkbride (1809-1883) Physician, advocate for the mentally ill and founder of the Association of Medical Superintendents of American Institutions for the Insane, a precursor to the American Psychiatric Association

Dr. Thomas Story Kirkbride was born to a family of Quaker farmers on July 31st 1809 in Bucks County, Pennsylvania. His father deemed him too frail for farming but, recognizing his intelligence and sensitivity, encouraged him to pursue a medical career. At age eighteen, after completing his primary education, he began to study medicine under the tutelage of Dr. Nicholas Bellevillein of Trenton, New Jersey, eventually being awarded a degree in medicine from the University of Pennsylvania in 1832.

Kirkbride wanted to be a surgeon

which was the most prestigious and lucrative specialty in medicine. However, he was unable to gain residency at the Pennsylvania Hospital in Philadelphia. Instead, through family connections, he was offered residency at the Quaker Friends Asylum for the Insane in Frankford, a small town on the outskirts of Philadelphia. Kirkbride accepted the position, not out of any particular interest in treating the insane, but as a springboard for his future at the Pennsylvania Hospital.

At 'Friends', Kirkbride observed and was impressed by the treatment afforded patients. Historically, the insane were considered incurable and were often chained to walls, unclothed, in a dungeon like environment. Friends Asylum was progressive for its time, establishing a family atmosphere, removing physical restraints, and providing the patients with stimulating mental and physical activities. Kirkbride applied himself thoroughly and his superiors at Friends wrote of the "faithful and exemplary discharge of his duties". Although his experience at Friends was rewarding and proved invaluable in his future endeavors, he still longed to be a surgeon. His wish was granted when, in March 1833, he was offered a residency at the Pennsylvania Hospital. Elated, Kirkbride accepted immediately and left for Philadelphia with no thoughts of ever returning to the treatment of the insane.

Kirkbrides performance at his new post was typically outstanding. He also nurtured a growing private practice which augmented his income. In both careers he was known for his kindness and compassion in treating patients, sane or otherwise. This did not go unnoticed. In 1840 the Hospital Governors, based mostly on his record at Friends, offered him the position of Superintendent at the newly built Pennsylvania Hospital for the Insane. Kirkbride accepted, again more for the prestige and financial security it offered than any personal desire to return to the treatment of the mentally ill. Yet, that is what he would do for the remaining 43 years of his life.

The new superintendent immersed himself in the world of the insane, collecting and devouring everything written on the treatment and housing of the mentally ill. It was the buildings themselves that most interested him. He noticed aspects in the design of the new facility that he considered ill planned in regard to creating a restorative ambience and he began to envision a hospital environment that by its very design would have a curative effect on its inhabitants.

By the early 1850's the growing patient population was putting a strain on "Kirkbride's Hospital", as it had come to be known, giving Kirkbride the opportunity to realize his vision. He convinced the Hospital Governors to approve funds to build a new facility based on his theories. "The Kirkbride plan" was born and for the next several decades would influence the construction of some 300 mental asylums. Thomas Story Kirkbride himself would come to be known as the foremost authority on hospital design.

Kirkbride became a founding member of the Association of Medical Superintendents of American Institutions of the Insane and served as its president for eight years. In 1854 he published *On the Construction, and General Arrangements of Hospitals for the Insane*, which was quickly recognized as the definitive work on the subject and secured his reputation as one of the leading experts in the treatment of the mentally ill. (13)

The Kirkbride Plan

Thomas Kirkbride envisioned an asylum constructed around a central administration building flanked by two wings of tiered wards. This was his "linear plan" which segregated the male patients from the female and each wing had equal exposure to fresh air, natural light, and views of the farmland around the asylum from all sides. Each wing was sub-divided by "wards", the more disruptive patients were on the lower floors and the more rational were placed on the upper floors closer to the administration offices. The purpose of this concept was to stress a more natural environment as far from pollutants in the urban centers as possible. The impressively large campuses were landscaped or configured as farmland making the asylum as self-sufficient as possible; allowing some inmates to work the gardens as well, and then the produce was sold or consumed by the patients and staff. Patients were encouraged to participate in other chores as well as taking part in games and outdoor recreation, helping foster and maintain social skills. (14)

There were several Kirkbride buildings constructed in New York, many of which are chronicled here. Most were built between 1848 and 1890. Each group of buildings followed the same basic floor plan advocated by Kirkbride but different architects executed their own interpretation of the final rendering. In the United States, there are more than forty Kirkbride buildings in existence. The sheer immensity of the total number of buildings constructed and the size of the acreage purchased for each building's grounds is hard to comprehend, even by today's standards. However, toward the end of the nineteenth century, the Kirkbride Plan began to lose its prominence. For one, there was a lack of concrete evidence showing any increase in the number of permanently cured patients and secondly, there was no reduction in the number of patients in need of help. This eventually caused the mental healthcare establishment to seek alternate forms of treatment. A new generation of asylum superintendents advocated different types of designs for asylums based on different concepts of care. Eventually, the large state hospital concept became obsolete. (15)

Most Kirkbride buildings that still exist are deteriorating due to neglect. Many have been demolished because they are too expensive to renovate and the land they occupy is now more commercially valuable than the buildings themselves. They are rapidly vanishing, signally an end to a remarkable period in the history of mental health care. The buildings and the people who served in them and were served by them, the 'mad houses' of the day; shape the hidden history of insane asylums in 19th-century New York which we will now explore. (16)

Chapter 2
Belle Vue

As New York City grew to over 8,000 in population by 1731, the "vagabonds, lunatics and idle beggars" could not be ignored by the rest of society, and construction of a "Public Workhouse and House of Correction" was begun in 1735. The budget for this ambitious project was £80 and 50 gallons of rum. The building was ready for occupancy by early 1736, with an upper floor infirmary measuring about 25 by 23 feet that contained six beds. Dr.

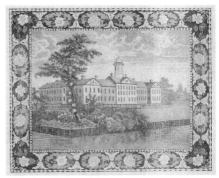

Bellevue Hospital founded in 1736 as a six bed almshouse hospital. Services included treating the insane.

John Van Beuren was appointed medical officer, at £100 a year, which included supplying all medications. Although it had no name as yet, Bellevue Hospital had been born. The rest of the building was also quite remarkable, as it included areas for hard labor, instruction in sewing, knitting, spinning, weaving and working in leather and iron. There was also an adjacent farm. This "occupational therapy" approach to the social problems of the day made this a poorhouse and correctional institution far ahead of its time.

The records are sparse until the time of the Revolutionary War, but periodic large expenses suggest alterations and additions. In 1776, when the city was occupied by the British, prison inmates were transferred to Poughkeepsie. It is known that large numbers of destitute and insane persons were admitted after a large fire on September 21, 1776. After the evacuation in 1783, the poor were brought back down the Hudson and several outbuildings had to be added to increase the capacity. Poor-taxes to support the alms house became a major burden at this time. (17)

Admissions Criteria

The following is a record of the poor and insane brought to Belle Vue in 1838. As can be ascertained, many admissions were for short periods. Reasons for admittance include; children becoming orphans as result of one or both parent's death (four cases), homelessness and destitution (three cases), insanity (three cases) and old-age coupled with a crippling disability such as blindness (four cases). Causes for patient's eventual disposition includes, death, discharge and transfer to other facilities including orphanages and Blackwell Island Lunatic Asylum. (18)

Annie Meyo, age 8, and her brother, Arthur, age 6
Born in Cohoes
Cause of dependence: Mother Dead, Father unable to provide for them
Father is of intemperate habits
Removed by relatives, Oct. 23, 1840

Maria Watts, age 65
Born in England
A housewife and a widow with temperate habits and a school education
has one child, in England
Cause of dependence: Old age & destitution

Daniel Hennessy, age 5
Born in Ireland
Cause of dependence: Made destitute by death of father
Will soon be removed to an orphan asylum.

Ellen Cahill, age 30
Born in Ireland
A woman of intemperate habits; unable to read or write
Cause of dependence: Insanity
Absconded Nov. 12, 1839

Jane Patterson, age 28
Born in Ireland
A woman of temperate habits; unable to read or write
Occupation: servant
She has one child
Cause of dependence: Blind

Ida Bartholomew, age 17
Born in Albany
Cause of dependence: Epilepsy
This child has been an epileptic for the last 10 years. Her father resides in this county in moderate circumstances, but has a helpless family. The mother died a few months previous to her entrance here.

William Lawlor, age 8
Born in New York
Cause of dependence: Homeless by death of parents

Honora Murphy, age 22
Born in Ireland
A woman of intemperate habits; can read
Occupation: servant
Has one child, who is supported by relatives
Cause of dependence: Sentenced 3 months for drunkenness
Died Oct. 20, 1839

Kate Southerland, age 32
Born in New Jersey
A woman of temperate habits; unable to read or write
Occupation: servant
Cause of dependence: Homeless & out of employment

John Fitzgerald, age 24
Born in Ireland
A laborer of intemperate habits; unable to read or write
Cause of dependence: Blindness & Insanity
This man has been blind during the past four years, during which time his reason has been failing. He is destructive and filthy in his person & habits. It cannot be ascertained that others of the family were insane.

Mary Harmon, age 47
Born in Ireland
A woman of temperate habits; can read and write
Occupation: servant
Cause of dependence: Unable to procure employment
Discharged Oct. 29, 1839

John Hutchinson, age 21
Born in Germany
A laborer of temperate habits; can read
Cause of dependence: Insanity
This young man was first admitted to the Insane Asylum in May 1834, and (illegible) under treatment about 6 months, where he was discharged … to his father. He was arrested in May 1838 for an attempt to rape, & again pronounced insane, & committed to the Insane Asylum, where will probably remain during life.

Annie Maxwell, age 65
Born in Ireland
A widow and housewife of temperate habits; unable to read or write
Cause of dependence: old age & destitution

Catherine Baker, age 24; came to the almshouse with her two children
Born in New York
A widow and housewife of temperate habits; unable to read or write
Cause of dependence: Made homeless by death of husband
This woman seems to be a respectable person. She will probably go out in a short time & provide for herself. She is both earnest & willing.
Discharged Oct. 9, 1839

Hugh Rourke, age 50
Born in Ireland
A laborer of intemperate habits; can read
Cause of dependence: Insanity
Re-admission in Insane Asylum. The physicians have no hope of his recovery.

New York would soon surpass Philadelphia in size and importance. The 1810 census listed a population of 96,373. Sanitation was almost non-existent; disease was rampant. Severe epidemics of yellow fever ravaged the city annually from 1794 to 1805; waterfront areas teemed with plague. Filth filled the streets and the sewers were but open canals. In 1807 the city began extensive municipal improvements and in 1811 it purchased six acres of the Kip's Bay Farm along the East River called Belle Vue Place, along one border, which already contained a building — the first to bear the name Belle Vue Hospital. It was used off and on while the city tried to cope with the persistent threat of yellow fever. A considerable proportion of the hospital staff was occupied in burying the dead. Belle Vue had established its own cemetery nearby in 1757 — this may well be another "first" among American hospitals.

New York's ambitious plans ran into a major snag in 1812, when the U.S. entered into war with Britain. It was not until 1814 that any progress was reported in construction and finally, in 1816, the buildings were open "to receive their guests." The buildings were built to last (perhaps they expected another British invasion), as they were constructed of gneiss rock from the immediate area. It was around this time that Belle Vue was first contracted to be named "Bellevue."(19)

The medical department was reorganized in 1800, with the appointment of a salaried officer to act as physician, surgeon, and accoucheur. Dr. William McIntosh served in this capacity for five years, at which time the medical staff was doubled and an apothecary was added. A second physician was rarely employed, until 1817 however, it was realized that one doctor could not care for over 200 hospitalized patients including the insane. Night calls and delivering babies became ever more frequent, and a house physician also had to prepare and administer all of the drugs prescribed by the visiting doctor. Staffing was now set at two visiting doctors and two interns.

Belle Vue

Disease Strikes back

Throughout the early part of the 19th century the hospital continued to expand in physical size and staffing in an attempt to cope with an ever-increasing case load which continued to include sporadic epidemics of yellow fever. Of the infectious diseases, typhus fever epidemics were by far the worst challenge, with a death rate of about one in 10.

In 1825 both resident physicians became ill with typhus; Dr. Belden died. He was but the first of many doctors to give their lives while on duty at Bellevue. By 1884, 27 house staff doctors had died from diseases contracted during their hospital service.

Predatory Politics

Thanks to political mishandling and exploitation, Bellevue Hospital endured a long period early in the 19th century that caused even the most loyal employees to desert. Controlled by inept political appointees, the mismanaged hospital became a shambles. The mortality rate increased to 20 percent and one year reached 33 percent. Conditions were pitiful, supplies had been plundered, the farm was neglected, and little food was available. In 1837, eight nurses and servants "escaped" from Bellevue, leaving the sick, the poor and the insane to fend for themselves. What drove them to this action? "The whole concern was filled with typhus from top to bottom. The patients were lying in their filthy blankets, destitute of sheets and pillow-cases, and in some chronic cases they had not had a change for three months....There was not even any Indian meal for poultices — no rags to dress the wounds."

Finally the commissioners took measures to improve the situation. Part of the solution was to free the hospital of the burdens of not only providing medical care, but caring for the mentally ill and also being a penal institution. Male prisoners were sent to a new penitentiary on Blackwell's Island. Smallpox patients soon followed. Female prisoners were sent to the Tombs, and the lunatics were removed to a new asylum, also on Blackwell's Island. It took 10 more years before the alms house was also removed. By mid-century, Bellevue had a new board comprised of the most distinguished physicians and surgeons in New York, and the institution began to assume its rightful role in the community of medical care.

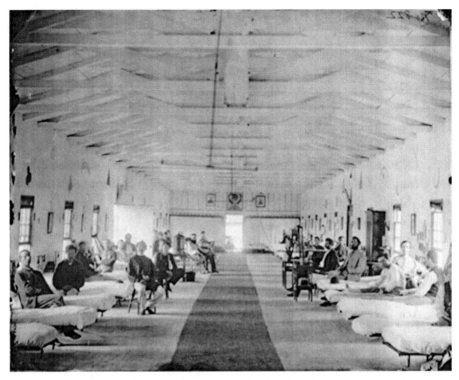

Bellevue would eventually become New York's flagship health and psychiatric care delivery system and one of the Nation's largest hospitals. Bellevue currently handles nearly 500,000 outpatient clinic visits, 145,000 emergency visits and some 26,000 inpatients yearly.

Bellevue Hospital Today

Eventually Bellevue Hospital would become one of the largest public hospitals in the United States. Today the hospital handles over 500,000 outpatient visits, 140,000 emergency room visits, and 26,000 inpatients a year. (20)

Chapter 3

The Lunatic Asylum on Blackwell Island

In 1693, dozens of "witches" were barbarically put to death in colonial Massachusetts, a shameful episode of mass hysteria overtaking otherwise "sensible" citizens. It is a good bet that quite a few of those who were hanged or pressed to death were, in some way, mentally unstable. In any event, the Salem Witch Trials offer a glimpse of attitudes towards mental illness, at the end of the 17th century.

In the last few generations, society has adopted a more enlightened attitude towards the mentally ill, giving it equal status to "physical" diseases in terms of insurance coverage and medical treatment options. Yet, anyone who has walked the "mental wards" of big-state hospitals will no doubt feel some mixture of depression and shock at the lamentable conditions often present. Even the best intentions can fall flat when faced with economic realities. (21)

New York Builds an Asylum

Such is the story of the New York City Lunatic Asylum on Blackwell's (now Roosevelt) Island, a small two-mile spit of land in the East River just off Manhattan. What started as a noble attempt to provide shelter to "lunatics" and the poor, degenerated into a national scandal that was uncovered by the intrepid and quite beautiful reporter, Nellie Bly, more about Nellie later.

What is known today as Roosevelt Island was first named Hog Island when it was purchased from the Canarsie Indians in 1637 by the Dutch

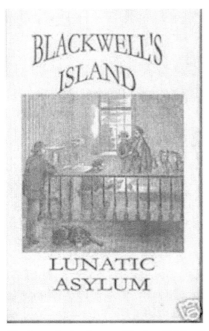

The Lunatic Asylum at Blackwell Island was established in 1839. Part of the asylum was destroyed by fire in 1859 and was rebuilt. It closed permanently in 1895.

Governor of New Amsterdam. The island became English property after the Dutch were defeated in 1666 and eventually passed to Robert Blackwell in 1686. Jump ahead to 1796, and we see Robert Blackwell's great grandson, Jacob, constructing Blackwell House on the island, which remains today a sterling example of period architecture.

New York City purchased the island in 1828 and proceeded to build a penitentiary there four years later. Soon thereafter, designer Alexander Jackson Davis was commissioned to design a Gothic Revival structure known as "The Octagon". Davis was a native New Yorker who studied art and design under the influence of the noted architect Josiah Brady. The Octagon was a five-story, eight-sided building that used locally-mined stone. It was designed in 1834 to serve as the main entrance to the New York City Lunatic Asylum, which at the time was one of the first mental asylums in the country. The building erected by the City, in 1839, was a scaled-back version of the elaborate plans drawn up by Davis. The original plans had called for a pair of matching rotundas, but that design was not economically feasible.

The Lunatic Asylum was one of several public houses that were built on Blackwell's Island in the 19th century, including a, penitentiary, workhouse, and hospital.(22)

Early Conditions

The idea for establishing the Lunatic Asylum grew out of the intolerable conditions then extant at Bellevue Hospital in Manhattan. A few crowded

The Lunatic Asylum on Blackwell Island

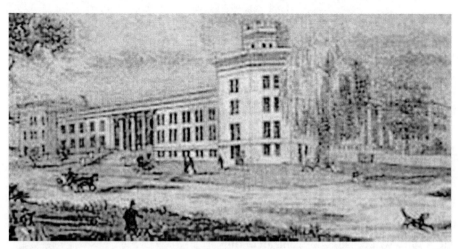

Thousands of the cities mentally ill were admitted to the asylum between 1839 and 1895 and the press and public's fascination grew intense during those years.

and ill-kept wards served as the confinement area for the city's severely disturbed residents. A slow liberalization of the public's attitudes towards the mentally ill brought the city to consider treatment as an alternative to simple confinement. But it would be wrong to overstate how quickly attitudes changed. After its opening in 1841, the Asylum's patients were initially supervised by inmates from the nearby penitentiary, under the guidance of a small staff of physicians.

The conditions of treatment in these early years were apparently so abysmal that the medical staff revolted and forced the City to hire nurses and orderlies. In 1850, Medical treatment was expanded to include physical activities and occasionally, entertainment. Patients were allowed to do useful work: men could tend the local vegetable gardens or work on constructing sea walls to increase the land available on the island; women were expected to perform chores such as sewing and housekeeping. Private citizens and publishing companies contributed funds and books to create a library. There were also weekly dances and even a billiard table.

The Asylum was, however, not a pleasant place by any stretch of the imagination. Funds were tight and there was a good deal of overcrowding. Food was inadequate and the Asylum's inmates often suffered from diseases such as cholera and typhus. Still, some efforts were made to improve their lot. Buildings were added to relieve some of the overcrowding, and this allowed the violent patients to be separated from the others. By 1875, things had improved enough that a reporter for a Harper's weekly proclaimed the facility "healthy and convenient". This, however, turned out to be an overstatement. (23)

Nellie Bly

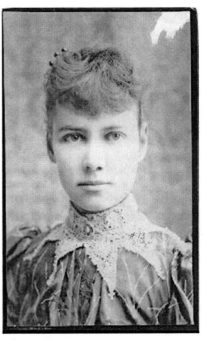

Elizabeth Jane Cochrane took the pen name Nellie Bly when she decided to break into the male-dominated world of journalism. She talked her way into a reporting job at the Pittsburgh Dispatch in 1880, where she concentrated on "women's topics" like theater and the arts. She gradually tired of reporting exclusively on such fluff. Bly moved on to New York in 1887 where, after four starving months, she landed a job at the New York World, the newspaper owned by James Pulitzer. The terms of her employment demanded that she secretly infiltrate the Lunatic Asylum and reveal whether ongoing reports of neglect and brutality were actually true.

Elizabeth Cochrane, aka Nellie Bly (1864-1922) feigned insanity in order to be admitted to Blackwell Island in order to write an expose. Her book, Ten Days in a Mad-House, was responsible for significant mental health reforms.

This meant, of course, that Nellie would have to convincingly feign madness, something she felt next to impossible. But Nellie was nothing if not game and so she signed on to the job. She prepared for the role by checking into a rooming house, staying awake all night and acting paranoid. She was arrested the next day and feigned amnesia in front of the judge, who concluded she was on drugs. Doctors declared her insane and untreatable – "a hopeless case" – and she was then committed to the Asylum. Local papers, including the New York Times, ran stories about the vacant-eyed waif who couldn't remember anything.

The Lunatic Asylum on Blackwell Island

Nellie recounted the Asylum conditions in her report, "Ten Days in a Mad-House". The food was horrible, the drinking water was dirty, violent patients were tied by ropes, and patients were forced to sit on cold benches all day long. Cold bathwater, wandering rats, abusive nurses and physical beatings all added to the misery. Nellie wrote that the treatment was perfect for creating insanity but not very good for curing it. The following is a short excerpt describing her misery: "...My teeth chattered and my limbs were ... numb with cold. Suddenly, I got three buckets of ice-cold water...one in my eyes, nose and mouth."

After ten days of undercover sleuthing, The World arranged for Nellie's release. Her report which would later became a best-selling book, caused a national sensation and led directly to a grand jury investigation into conditions of the Asylum. Bly even acted as tour director for the jury when they visited the Asylum to see for themselves how the place was run. The trip was supposed to be a surprise, but somehow the Asylum management got tipped off about an hour in advance. The nurses offered contradictory stories, but one of the doctors was more forthcoming – he agreed the food was poor and the baths were cold, but blamed it all on lack of funds. He also could offer no defense of the nurses against the charge of cruelty and went on to question the competency of several of the doctors.

To her surprise, the grand jury agreed with Nellie, and called for a budget increase to address the problems that Nellie had so dutifully reported. The Department of Public Charities and Corrections increased its funding by $850,000 and agreed to a series of reforms suggested by Nellie, including one for more thorough oversight. Nellie went on to other great things and died at age 57. She was inducted into the National Women's Hall of Fame in 1968. (24)

***

Then, as now, the number of indigent "insane" people in New York threatened to overwhelm the city's resources, and by 1894, plans went forward to transfer inmates of the Asylum to various hospitals on newly-acquired Ward Island, another small island in the East River. The Asylum was renamed Metropolitan Hospital and became a treatment center for patients with tuberculosis. By the 1950s, the buildings on (now) Roosevelt Island were abandoned for a couple of decades. When New York State threatened to demolish The Octagon, the

Landmarks Preservation Commission came to its rescue, although the side-wings were torn down. The commission referenced an 1865 report from Dr. R.L. Parsons, who was the resident doctor at the Lunatic Asylum at the time, that the Octagon "has symmetry, a beauty and grandeur even, that is to be admired." Visitors today can still enjoy the aesthetic beauty of Octagon, even if they are ignorant of its dark history. (25)

Perhaps future generations will look back at the way we treated the mentally disturbed during our own time with a mix of astonishment and horror, just as we do now when we recollect the Lunatic Asylum on Blackwell's Island.

Chapter 4

Monroe County Insane Asylum

Like most of the mental institutions built during the mid-19th century, the Monroe County Insane Asylum in Rochester, New York, began with good intentions and altruistic motives. In 1826, the Monroe County Alms House was created to house and care for the area's growing poor and indigent population. At this time, the mentally ill poor were grouped together with the non-mentally ill poor. Impoverished people from Monroe County suffering from various hardships all lived together at the Alms House, with the stated purpose of the Alms House being to take care of "the raving maniac, the young child, the infirm old man, and the seducer's victim". A penitentiary was also built on the same grounds. While the intentions of the creators of

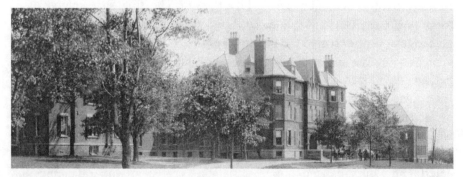

In 1824, Monroe County founded its first poorhouse to care for "the raving maniac, the young child, the infirm old man, and the seducers victim".

these facilities were no doubt noble, having all of society's "undesirables" sequestered away in one location without attention to their very different individual needs and problems was less than ideal.

At this time the mentally ill at the Alms House did not receive specialized treatment, being rather lumped together with everyone else, but this would soon change. By 1857, changing societal attitudes toward the mentally ill began leading to the creation of residential homes for the mentally ill across the country. The directors of the Alms House decided to add a special wing that was specifically dedicated to the insane. While still considered a part of the Alms House, the wing was given its own name- the Monroe County Insane Asylum. This separation, of course, also benefited the other, non-mentally ill inmates of the Alms House, particularly the children, since some of the mentally ill patients were considered violent. The wing for the mentally ill soon became overcrowded, with the patients living for a while in cramped and deplorable conditions. A few years later, in 1862, the number of Alms House residents being admitted into the mental asylum wing had increased so significantly that they now required their own separate building. The establishment of the large new building helped to improve conditions dramatically. (26)

Life at the Monroe County Insane Asylum

For the first decade or so of its existence, the Monroe County Insane Asylum earned a positive reputation, becoming known as a place where the mentally ill were treated humanely and with dignity. The first superintendent of Monroe County Insane Asylum, Dr. Lord, was considered to be a kind and gentle person who treated the patients very well. Patients were intentionally kept busy, active and occupied, which was thought to be therapeutic. The patients developed a sense of purpose and usefulness, and were distracted from their troubles, by engaging in housework around the asylum, as well as landscaping and farm work on the surrounding grounds. An emphasis was placed on a plain but nutritious and wholesome diet, as well as physical exercise. They were also allowed and encouraged to participate in more entertaining pursuits and hobbies, such as crafts, artwork, dancing and music. Instruction was even given in intricate textile arts such as weaving and embroidery, and this seemed to significantly benefit some of the patients.

Monroe County Insane Asylum

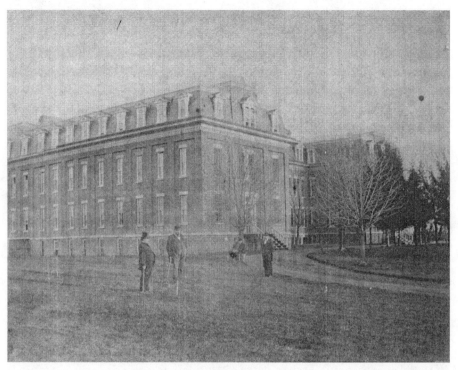

In 1891 Monroe County Insane Asylum became Rochester State Hospital. Instructions of rug weaving, washing & ironing, and judging by this photo, croquet, were used as therapies.

During this time the asylum was also known to be neat, orderly and an overall pleasant to live.

By the 1870's, the Monroe County Insane Asylum began to be plagued by the problems that were increasingly common at the well-intended mental institutions across the nation. As it became more and more socially acceptable for the mentally ill to be sent to residential asylums instead of locked away in family attics or basements, the asylums grew proportionally more crowded. Monroe County Insane Asylum was no exception, and so by the 1870's had grown overcrowded and decidedly less pleasant. With too many patients for the staff to handle, gentle and humane treatment and individual attention was no longer the norm, and the patients at the asylum came to sometimes be treated more like prisoners than well cared for residents.

Changes in 1890

In 1890, after a few decades of increasing interest in long-term treatment for the mentally ill, New York State passed the State Care Act, which allowed for the establishment and financial backing of state-funded mental institutions. Under this act, the State of New York offered to purchase and operate the Monroe County Insane Asylum. The state purchased the asylum for $50,000 in 1891 and renamed it the Rochester State Hospital. At this time, Eugene Henry Howard, a graduate of the University of Buffalo Medical Department, became superintendent of the asylum. He remained in his supervisory role at the asylum for 35 years. After the purchase of the asylum, the state spent additional funds in order to renovate and expand the hospital, to provide space for more patients and to help counteract the overcrowding issue. Over the ensuing years, the hospital regularly added more beds- and where necessary, buildings- but expansion could not keep up with increasing patient numbers. The hospital continued to face overcrowding issues at various times throughout much of its existence. (27)

Later Years

The Rochester State Hospital has been in continual use over the years, serving the more serious mental health needs of the Rochester area. In the 1970's it was renamed once again, from the Rochester State Hospital to the Rochester Psychiatric Hospital. The psychiatric hospital still exists today, as a large state-funded treatment facility, which continues to offer residential treatment for both adolescents and adults. The local sheriff's office also has a forensics department on the premises. (28)

The Remember Garden

While the original intentions of the founders of the Monroe County Insane Asylum, and similar institutions around the country, were lofty, there was a definite ugly side to such places. The Alms House and later the asylum provided a home and care for many of Rochester's most vulnerable citizens- the poor, the mentally disabled, and those abandoned by their families of all ages. The Monroe County Insane Asylum was a safe haven for many, but even within this safe haven the poor and mentally ill were without status or power. When the residents died, they became nameless, anonymous and probably went un-mourned.

In 1984 a large mass grave was discovered in Highland Park in Rochester, New York, when a bulldozer which was being used in a terracing project uncovered very old human remains. The mysterious grave was marked by a single large stone, without any inscriptions or names. Researchers soon discovered that the dead men, women, and children who were buried here in this large, anonymous grave, were most likely patients from the Monroe County Insane Asylum who died in the 19th century. More than 700 individuals were buried in this mass grave, in simple and cheap wooden coffins, with no records being kept of the dead.

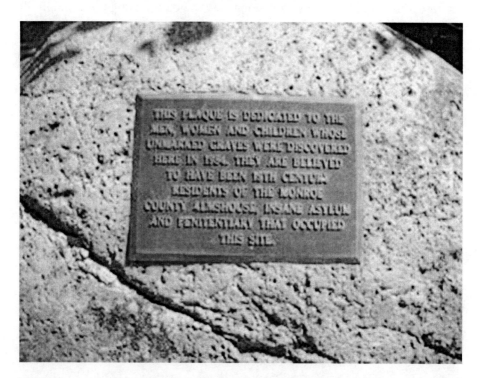

The Remember Garden. Over 700 unmarked graves from the original Monroe County Asylum were discovered in 1984. 305 bodies were interred at Mount Hope Cemetery along with this memorial.

In 2004, a living garden memorial called the Remember Garden was created at the site of the mass grave. The garden was established in order to honor the dead and provide them with the dignity they were denied at the time of their deaths. The garden is maintained by DePaul Community Services, and is crisscrossed by peaceful paths and benches where one can sit and reflect while surrounded by lilies, lilacs, pansies, shrubs and trees. The Remember Garden is a place to come and pay respects to those who died at the Monroe County Insane Asylum so many years ago.

The dead were those unfortunate enough to be born with mental illness or disability or in some cases something as minor as a seizure disorder, which at the time was enough to classify someone as mentally ill. While the Monroe County Insane Asylum and similar institutions represented a step in the right direction, there was still a long way to go in treating the mentally ill with dignity and humanity. 19th century residential mental institutions were certainly more humane than simply locking away the mentally ill in a basement and pretending they didn't exist, but were nonetheless limited in many ways. The patients were still seen by many as less than human and lacking individual worth or value, as evidenced by the way they were treated after death.

The Remember Garden is intended not only as a place to honor these specific dead, but also as a place to reflect soberly on the history of mental health treatment, how far it has come, and how much there is left to accomplish. Another major purpose of the Remember Garden is to motivate visitors to help remove the stigma attached to mental illness. The graves are no longer unmarked, instead decorated by a simple plaque asking visitors to remember those poor souls who died at the Monroe County Insane Asylum so long ago. While the founders, doctors, nurses and superintendents at the Monroe County Insane Asylum and other such institutions did the best they could with the knowledge they had at the time, the Remember Garden reminds us that life for the mentally ill in the 19th century was uncertain and difficult. (29)

Chapter 5
Rolling Hills

J ust before Christmas in the year 1826, an official announcement was made
in reference to a meeting of the Genesee County Board of Supervisors
in Bethany in order to establish a county poorhouse. More often than not
those in need of a county poorhouse were the orphaned, destitute elderly,
physically handicapped, or those judged to be insane. They were supervised by
representatives of the local community which oversaw the support and housing
of needy persons of all ages. Institutions of this kind were commonplace in the
United States during the first half of the 19th century. (30)

The Poorhouse

A large multi-story brick building, originally a stagecoach tavern, located near
the Bethany Center and Raymond Roads, was chosen as the best location for the
poorhouse, it also happened to be the exact geographical center of the county
at that time. On December 9, 1826, the following announcement appeared in
the Batavia Times newspaper:

"Notice is hereby given that the Genesee County Poorhouse will be ready
for the reception of paupers on the first day of January, 1827. The Overseers
of the Poor of the several towns of the County of Genesee are requested, in all
cases of removal of paupers to the county poorhouse, to send with them their
clothing, beds, bedding and such other articles belonging to the paupers as may
be necessary and useful to them."

The categories of persons who were considered eligible for admission, were habitual drunkards, lunatics (one who by disease, grief, or accident lost the use of reason or from old age, sickness, or weakness was so weak of mind as to be incapable of governing or managing their own affairs), state paupers (one who is blind, lame, old, or disabled with no income source) or vagrants.

The next year, in 1828, the county constructed a stone building which was attached to the poorhouse expressly for the confinement of "lunatics" and also for paupers who had been committed due to misconduct. Those declared "insane" were also housed at the County Home until late 1887 when the Board of Supervisors voted to send persons "suffering with acute insanity" elsewhere in the state.

The Farm

The poorhouse, known as the Genesee County Poor Farm or The County Home, was also a self-sufficient working farm, spanning over 200 acres, providing fuel and food for the entire establishment. The actual cost per person was very low, amounting to about $1.08 per week per resident. Many of the residents also crafted things to sell. The farm workers raised Holsteins, pigs, draft horses, chickens and ducks, vegetables and fruits and they canned jams, jellies, and meats. They also manned a bakery and a wood shop where coffins were made for use as needed and for sale to local mortuaries.

When an "inmate" grew old or very ill and died, the county buried those who had no family and the remaining records indicate there was once a cemetery on the property but there are no records that show where it was. At a meeting in 1886, the minutes state, "The burying ground we have improved by building a fence in front and grading and leveling the ground as much as could be done without injury to the graves."

As time passed and the grave stones crumbled, the cemetery's location became obliterated by roots, weeds, grass, and forest. No one tended the graves and all who died there were forgotten. A burial plot map has yet to be discovered but many still hope there is one to be found.

On June 6, 2004, five headstones dated from 1887 to 1888 were returned to the County and a memorial site was created for their permanent resting place. The Genesee County Historians dedicated a historical marker honoring those who died while living in the home from 1827 until it closed in 1974. (31)

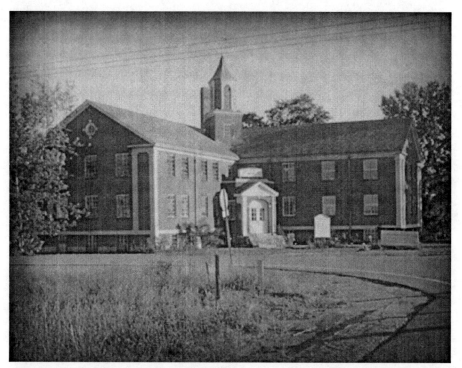

Rolling Hills, originally named, The Genesee County Poor Farm was founded in 1826. In 1828 a stone building was constructed attached to the poor house for the confinement of lunatics.

The Haunting

Since the closing of the Rolling Hills Asylum, the interest in evidence of paranormal activity has attracted considerable attention. The vacant red brick building, estimated at over 55,000 square feet of living space, is said to echo with the heartache and desolation of the insane that lived there through the years. The huge building still looms on the empty land, defiantly outliving most everything in sight, including the local residents. The decorative cupola sits atop the soaring roof and many of the windows of the dormers are broken, adding to the spookiness of the sprawling edifice. Periodically, paranormal experts have attempted to record and film any "ghosts" still lurking in the corners.(32) The hallways are like stop-still photography, with gurneys paused en route and an empty walker standing hesitantly as if waiting for its owner.

The kitchen seems prepared for dinner guests, the banging of pots and pans and the hiss of steam from the kettle, the floors still gleam in sections, almost whispering by themselves without the squeaky whistles of the nurse's shoes. The echoes of groans and sighs are sibilant in the psychiatric wing and the silence seems louder as the sunlight fades and there is no electricity to pop beams of light into the darkest corners. The curious and the eager will continue to explore the evidence of so many hurting souls who lingered here much too long. Some people have no doubts whatsoever that there are many spirits here of people who don't want to be gone... not just yet. Something keeps them strolling down the halls, checking in on their neighbors, straightening a draw sheet just so, shoving a wheelchair out of the way, watching the rain pepper the inside windowsill, sitting on one of the concrete garden benches by the growing vegetable garden, and waiting, waiting, waiting for the spring rain.

Rolling Hills Asylum remembers the babies and the children, the destitute, the elderly and the mad who lived their final days at the asylum. Their permeating sadness has taken root in the peeling paint and the crumbling mortar, soon to be forever suspended in each tremulous raindrop clinging to the tree branches.

Eventually, the recycling begins.

Chapter 6

Cattaraugus County Stone House

In 1824, the State Legislature of New York enacted a law requiring each county in the state to establish a county poor house. The local county legislatures were to purchase up to 200 acres of land to build these poor houses, with the building and maintenance costs to be paid by local taxes. In 1833, the County Legislature of Cattaraugus County, New York, voted to erect their county poor house in Machias to care for the county's insane, indigent, aged and orphaned. They took out local advertisements for land proposals.

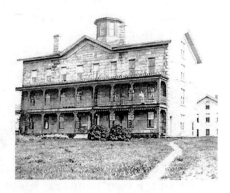

The Stone House of Cattaraugus County was established in 1837 to care for the indigent, aged, orphaned, infirm and insane.

The land where the Stone House Insane Asylum was established was purchased from Willard Jefferson in 1834. He sold his farm for $2300 and then moved to Ohio. The land consisted of 200 acres and construction began immediately on a number of wood frame buildings to house the patients. Throughout the latter half of the 19th century, the land served as a residence and a self-sufficient farm to those who were placed there. (33)

The wood frame structures were completed by 1835 and housed 33 paupers. Just a decade later, fire destroyed the main structure, including all of the books and records for the facility. New structures were quickly built.

The need for proper housing was evident when, in 1857, a committee formed by the state Senate paid a visit to the poor house. They found the conditions to be unacceptable. Of the two structures they looked at, one was very old and let in the chilly winter air. It had an obvious loose construction and was in a state of decay. It was also very filthy. The second structure on the property was newer, but still not well constructed, which made it un-inhabitable. The following are their conclusions:

The Yates Report

This is an old and dilapidated building of wood and brick, erected in 1832, in size thirty-two by ninety-six, with a wing, twenty-four by sixty feet, aside from these is a small building for the insane; attached is a farm of one hundred and sixty acres, yielding a revenue of $2,000.There are no basements. The rooms are warmed by stoves, but are without means of ventilation. The number of inmates was fifty-six; forty males, sixteen females. Of these forty-six are native born, ten foreign, and seven under sixteen years of age. The sexes are separated only at night; they are under two keepers, male and female. In one room as many as thirty-two persons were placed. The inmates are supported at a weekly cost of forty-four cents. The paupers are employed on the farm and about the house. The house has not been visited during the year by supervisors. It is supplied with Bibles; through no provision is made for religious instruction they often have service on the Sabbath. A common school is taught in the house during six or eight months of the year. The fare of the paupers is plain and wholesome and supplied by the keeper. For medical attendance a physician is called when needed and paid per visit. During the year there have occurred six births and seventeen deaths. They have no pest house.

Of the inmates twelve are lunatics; six males, and six females; all are paupers and six of them have been treated at the State asylum. They have no particular medical attendance. A small wooden building, size twenty-six by forty feet, has recently been erected for their accommodation, though hardly fitted for its designed purpose. The cells are small, illy ventilated and constructed of rough hemlock boards and plank, in which the lunatics are confined with no bedding but straw, and an insufficient supply of clothing. The building is so open that it is impossible properly to warm it in winter. Four are confined in cells. They are also sometimes restrained by the "mittens". The construction of the house is such as to allow classification; the power of discharge is exercised

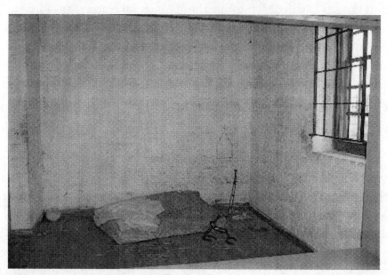

In a 1857 report, the living conditions of the 'inmates' was found to be, dilapidated, cold in the winter and offensive from accumulated filth.

by the superintendents. Application has been made
during the year, for admission to the Utica asylum
in six cases, and as often refused. The lunatics
sometimes escape and are never again heard from.
Ten of the paupers are idiotic, all males. There
is one blind. Two-thirds are brought here through
intemperance. (34)

Once the report was issued, authorization for more land and construction
of a new building were approved. A report by L.S. Jenks, L.D. Warner and
William Napier concluded that a main building needed to be constructed. It
was to be built by November 1861 and not exceed the cost of $12,000.

The Stone House

In 1860, the County Supervisors commissioned to have the Machias Stone
House built. It was to serve as the centerpiece of the Cattaraugus County
Alms-House and Insane Asylum, which later became the Cattaraugus County
Home Farm and Infirmary. It is the only building of the original complex of
four buildings that still survives. In 1868, Mr. John Napier was hired to build
the house. He was well known in the community as a local stone cutter,
building the Samuel Butler home in Machias and the Ten Broeck Academy
in Franklinville. Some of Napier's national projects included the Old State
Capital building in Springfield, IL, the bridge spanning the Mississippi River
at St. Paul, MN and the dam across the Merrimac River in Lawrence, MA.
(35)

Construction

The Napier family quarry was the source of the stone used to build the Stone
House. The structure originally stood four floors tall with a pitched roof
and a cupola, built in a Gothic style. Due to roof problems in the 1950s,
the top floor and cupola were removed. The total cost of building the Stone
House came to $18,000. It accommodated 100 people, plus the keeper and
his family.

Cattaraugus County Stone House

The building of the Stone House was completed in 1868. In 1869, the property had 60 people including one mute, one blind person, 23 insane and six children. The older buildings on the property were to be abandoned.

By 1878, the farm was still not self-sufficient, but during the 1890s, it was the patients and county employees who helped to create an example of self-reliance with poultry, meat and dairy products from the barn as well as fruit and vegetables from the orchards and gardens on the property. According to an 1893 biography of the county, the alms-house farm was one of most productive farms in the county. Improvements to the structures and add-ons were constructed as the population grew.

North of the Stone House a cemetery was established for those who had no funds or family members to inter them in another cemetery in the county. At least 123 former patients are buried there.

While the county's poor house was self-sufficient due to the labor of the patients, it was still an insane asylum. During the 19th century, standards for these facilities often resembled prisons rather than healthcare facilities and were notoriously lacking in care. According to an 1881 study of the indoor pauper published in The Atlantic Monthly, residents of county poor houses were often chained in dungeon-like rooms, insufficiently cared for and left in hot, filthy environments for extended periods of time. The study focused on the poor house of Onondaga County, but stated that its condition was comparable to the conditions found in Alleghany and Cattaraugus counties. This study did point out that facilities with full time physicians and well paid employees were less likely to carry out such abuses. (36)

John Little

The superintendant of the Cattaraugus County almshouse (Stone House) in the late 1880's was John Little Jr., former Sheriff of Cattaraugus County. Little is largely credited with helping to improve the lives of the inmates and patients in his charge by employing more staff and supplementing the income of the institution with proceeds from farming and wood working as noted above. Little would also become engaged in his previous role as Sheriff, in one of the most notorious episodes in county history, captured in lurid detail in this New York Times article.

The New York Times, Dec., 3, 1888

FINISHING THE CARPET SHE HAD BEEN WEAVING BECAME MRS. CLARKE'S FINISH

Martha Marble of Farmersville was only about 16 years old when she married Charles Clarke, 26, in 1878. Charles worked on the same large farm that Martha's family did but their homes were "about 30 rods" apart.

In the autumn of 1883, after having endured five years of marriage, she left Charles because, "he was a drinking, worthless fellow." When she left, Martha returned to her father's house nearby, taking many household furnishings with her. A few days later Martha returned with her brother to pick up a carpet that she was in the process of quilting. Since she was not quite done with it she decided to stay and finish the job.

Shortly thereafter, Charles came into the house and waited as she wove the carpet. After two hours, Martha's brother had to step away for a few minutes to tend to some cows. When he returned, he saw Clarke heading into nearby woods and found Martha mortally shot and stabbed. There were choke marks around her neck too. Later investigation indicated that after fleeing the bloody scene, Clarke ran to his own father's house about a mile away in Lyndon where he changed clothes. The

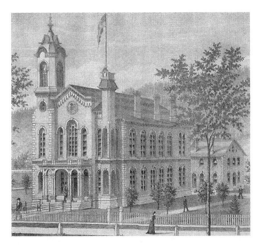

Little Valley Court House where trial of Charles Clarke was held. He would later be hanged for the crime.

blood-stained ones were found still wet from unsuccessful efforts to wash them clean.

Clarke was arrested at his father's house in Lyndon Dec. 7 by Sheriff John Little Jr.. Just before his capture, Clarke had attempted to cut his own throat, "but the wound was not fatal."

Cattaraugus County Stone House

Charles went to trial, and in short order was found guilty and sentenced to be hanged. About 100 invited guests witnessed the execution. The sheriff's wife and her friends watched from the second floor of the jail. The gallows was borrowed from another county and employed a weight instead of a trap door. (37)

TODAY

Currently, the original 1868 rebuilt Stone House is a fully functional, handicapped-accessible building utilized by the Cattaraugus County Department of Nursing Homes & the Dept. of Health, and is open to the public. As the oldest continually operated County building, and indeed the only County owned landmark left, the Stone House is a remarkable survivor to a by-gone era. (38)

Chapter 7

Albany Almshouse

S ome were alcoholics. Some
were mentally ill. Some were
criminals. And some had simply
fallen on hard times.

Mary Barker, a single woman
who emigrated from County
Clare, Ireland, came to the Albany
almshouse in February 1871
because she was too sick to support
herself. She died the following
December and was buried on the
almshouse grounds. She was 45.

Archaeologists don't know if
Mary Barker's body is among the

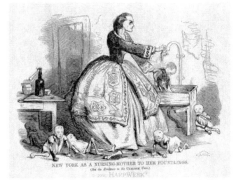

NEW YORK AS A NURSING-MOTHER TO HER FOUNDLINGS.

Established in 1826, the Albany Almshouse
would remain open for the next 100 years serving the most poor including their children and
the mentally ill of Abany county.

more than 1,000 remains excavated from the land of the old Albany almshouse.
Without a cemetery map to pinpoint where people were buried, researchers
have been unable to match any of the remains with names.

From 1826 to 1926, the New Scotland Avenue almshouse and its adjacent
cemetery served Albany's poorest and most mentally ill residents. In the years
since, the 116-acre site has been subdivided and put to various uses such as a
National Guard armory, a school, a laboratory for the state Health Department.

Construction crews occasionally found small sections of the old cemetery.

Albany Almshouse

When plans were announced for a $60 million medical research center on a vacant portion of the old almshouse site, researchers at first expected to find 200 bodies.

They found more than 1,000.

All are now being reburied at the Albany Rural Cemetery. When that process is completed, a memorial service will be held and a monument will be erected as a tribute to the people buried there.

"The intent would be to recognize these folks that are buried as individuals, to give them the respect accorded the dead," said Robert Lindsay, spokesman of the Charitable Leadership Foundation. The foundation, which is building the medical center, paid $1.7 million for the archaeological work.

"Archaeologists tend to take bones and keep them," Lindsay said. "We wanted to make sure that the scientists were able to study them and generate some useful scientific information… but then we wanted the remains removed to the cemetery for reburial.

Almshouses typically were government-run homes for people who couldn't support themselves or judged insane with no other housing alternatives. Intake records from the late 19th-century, on file at the New York State Archives, give some sense of the circumstances that forced people to come to the Albany almshouse. (39)

Margaret Coffee was 30 when she came to America in 1850, the daughter of an Irish farmer. She was unable to read or write and worked as a seamstress until the age of 48. Deteriorating eye-sight made it impossible for her to continue work and support herself.

"This woman is honest, sober, and industrious," the intake report reads. "She supported herself for a number of years after her husband's death. Being afflicted with sore eyes, she was compelled to seek admission here."

It's not clear from the records what happened to Margaret Coffee. The almshouse didn't begin to keep track of burials until 1878.

We do know the names of some of the later burials, names such as Kennedy, Burns, Campbell, Hamilton, and Cindillo. They were black and white, old and young. Some were insane, crippled or senile. And some were babies, stillborn to women living at the almshouse or dead within their first year.

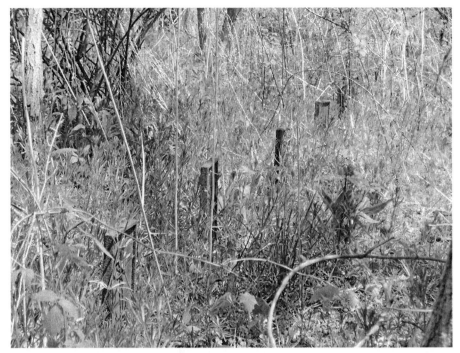

In 2001 archeologists unearthed approximately 1000 skeletons buried in unmarked graves at the site of the former Albany Almshouse. In some cases caskets were layered five and six deep.

Unmarked Graves

Those buried on almshouse grounds were the unclaimed poor of the region-those who died at the almshouse and those who died on the streets or at the nearby prison.

The Albany almshouse opened in 1826 on a farm then on the outskirts of the city. As with most almshouses of the era, a cemetery for burying the poor was part of the operation. But as with most almshouses, it lay largely forgotten, with no fences or headstones to serve as reminders of its burials.

"It's somewhat offensive that we didn't even know they were there," said archaeologist Louise Basa, president of the New York Archaeological Association.

Albany isn't alone. Historians say there are dozens of unmarked and largely forgotten almshouse cemeteries across the state.

Albany Almshouse

Archaeologists from the New York State Museum, which is overseeing the Albany project, say their work has already yielded valuable information.

Studying the remains provides researchers a better understanding of the lives of poor people (and the mentally ill) in the late 19th century. "History books are full of the rich and famous, and the notorious," said Andrea Lain, an archaeologist with the New York State Museum. But she added they are largely silent on the lives of the poor and working class.

The archaeologists found coffins in some spots layered five and six deep. Researchers cleaned and measured the bones, counted teeth and sketched coffin positions.

Because the people were so poor, they took little in the way of material goods with them to their graves. Most were buried in shrouds.

Their bones, however, give more detailed information, revealing clear signs of disease, overwork, poor medical care, and, in some cases, violence.

There were people with broken bones that never healed properly, some with anemia and rickets but just nine with signs of tuberculosis. "Tuberculosis was very common in the late 19th century," said state museum bio-archeologist Martin Solano. "However, the rib bones we need to make that determination just weren't there."

Demographics

In terms of demographics, archaeologists found many infants and people in their 20's and 30's.

"That's common with an early industrial population, with lots of infections and poor medical care," Solano said.

At least one-third of the bodies showed signs of serious infection, but the infections hadn't killed them. There was also lots of arthritis, even among people in their 30's. Teeth, even in young people, showed signs of exceptional wear and evidence of heavy pipe smoking, the cheapest way to smoke tobacco at the time. In 30 percent of the women and 40 percent of the men, semi-circular dips had been worn into teeth at the spot where a pipe might have been clenched.

Four women had notches in their teeth that researchers believe are linked to regularly pulling thread through their teeth, common among seamstresses.

One man's skull was shaped like a big bullet, a congenital abnormality that would have given a very unusual head shape during life.

Unique among the 894 burials was one coffin made of cast iron, with a glass viewing window at its head. The women died soon after her 40th birthday. She was about 5 feet, 2 inches.

"There was nothing to indicate who she was," Lain said, adding that researchers can only speculate that her family came forth upon her death and paid for the special casket.

Eventually, the New York State Museum in Albany will create an exhibit that will put some the archaeological findings into context. The exhibit may even give us a sense of what some of the people looked like. Museum researchers, using impressions taken from skulls, are attempting to reconstruct faces.

With the project nearing completion, historians said they'd like communities to make an effort to document unmarked burial yards. While federal legislation strictly protects American Indian burial areas, there are no similar protections for other graveyards.

Thomas Werner, the Albany city archeologist, said better local information about such sites would allow for planning. "The fact is there are bodies left and there's no notice of them. There are cars parked over them and any utility could dig through them. That bothers me," Werner said. (40)

Chapter 8

New York Lunatic Asylum at Utica

B y the mid-19th century, attitudes toward the mentally ill were beginning to change, and as these attitudes changed so did methods of dealing with the mentally ill members of society. Until this point the insane were mostly seen as something to be kept a family secret, the insane were locked away, hidden, and confined, with no thought toward treating their mental illness. If your family met with the misfortune of a mentally ill child or maiden aunt in the mid-1800's, you would most likely have locked them in your attic or cellar, bringing them food and water and hoping mostly to avoid calling embarrassing attention to your family. Mentally ill citizens without family support were commonly kept in jail cells or even the basements of public buildings. Insanity was seen by many as a permanent condition, rather than a treatable illness.

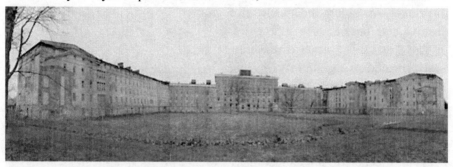

The Utica Insane Asylum was New York's first state-run facility designed to care for the mentally ill and one of the first in the United States.

Mid-19th century reforms, inspired by a spirit of altruistic activism as well as changes within the field of psychiatry itself, led to the creation of state-funded mental asylums throughout the U.S.. The first of these built in New York State was the New York State Lunatic Asylum, built in Utica in 1843. Like many of the early state-funded mental institutions, the New York State Lunatic Asylum was a large and architecturally impressive building surrounded by vast grounds and farmland. While some of the methods used at the New York State Lunatic Asylum and similar institutions can now be seen as inhumane and in some cases barbaric, the asylum was considered innovative at the time and was most likely created with the best of intentions.(41)

Dr. Amariah Brigham

The first superintendent and director at the New York State Lunatic Asylum was Dr. Amariah Brigham, a well-known and influential innovator in the field of psychiatry who helped give the asylum an air of prestige. Dr. Brigham was one of the founders of the Association of Medical Superintendents of American Institutions for the Insane, the earliest version of what would later become known as the American Psychiatric Association (APA). While serving as director at the asylum in Utica he also created and became the first editor of The American Journal of Insanity, later renamed to the more congenial The American Journal of Psychiatry.

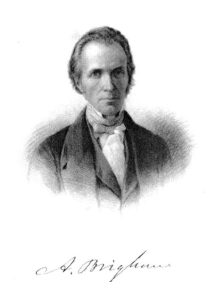

Dr. Amarah Brigham (1798-1949) Utica Asylums first director who became one of the original founders of the American Psychiatric Association.

Dr. Brigham was one of the first in the field of psychiatry to push for actual treatment of the mentally ill. At the New York State Lunatic Asylum, Dr. Brigham was able to implement many of his ideas for treatment. He believed that mental illness was often a result of poor environmental conditions, and therefore sought to create a wholesome and comforting environment at the asylum. Dr. Brigham placed a strong emphasis on the healing nature of quiet, solitude, and healthful activity. At the New York State Lunatic Asylum patients could enjoy nutritious food, large, airy rooms with wide windows that let in plenty of sunshine, exposure to fresh air and nature, and perhaps most importantly, vigorous physical exercise as well as mental activity. (42)

Treatment

This emphasis on physical health and useful activity was incredibly innovative at the time, because it assumed that mental illness was a state of unbalance or lack of health that could be treated and healed. While many of the particulars of Dr. Brigham's methods may seem primitive now, his overall attitude toward treating mental patients can be seen as humane, holistic and in some ways surprisingly modern. The patients at the New York State Lunatic Asylum helped maintain the grounds surrounding the asylum, which provided the patients with both physical exercise and a sense of purpose and usefulness. Dr. Brigham also set up a print shop at the asylum, where his psychiatric journal was printed with the help of industrious patients. While this can perhaps be viewed cynically as Dr. Brigham benefitting from the available free labor, keeping the patients busy with tasks that were actually helpful did genuinely comprise a significant part of his approach to treating the mentally ill.(43)

The Opal

The print shop at the New York State Lunatic Asylum served a unique purpose in addition to providing the patients with a job and printing copies of The American Journal of Insanity and this additional purpose was rather remarkable. The print shop was also where the asylum inmates printed their very own literary journal, The Opal, from 1850 until 1861. The Opal was published in ten volumes, and apparently distributed outside of the institution, at least in Utica. The journal included poetry, fictional prose, articles and essays, all written and edited by patients at the asylum. This provided the patients not only with another way to remain productive and occupied, but also with a serious creative outlet. Some of the common themes to emerge from the pages of The Opal include politics, human rights, liberty, insanity, and confinement. (44)

Harpers Ferry

Gerrit Smith was a well-known and respected 19th century abolitionist, philanthropist and social reformer. He was also one of the most famous, and perhaps unlikely, patients at the New York State Lunatic Asylum in Utica. A Utica native, Smith dedicated much of his life to the major progressive social causes of his day, including the abolition of slavery, the temperance movement, and the women's suffrage movement. In 1859 Smith became involved in the notorious Harpers Ferry incident through his friendship with fellow abolitionist John Brown, and this involvement ultimately led to his stay at the asylum in Utica.

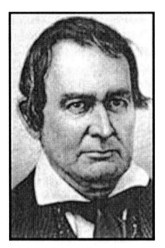

Gerrit Smith (1797-1874) Leading social reformer, abolitionist, politician and philanthropist. Was a member of the 'Secret Six', financially supporting John Browns raid at Harper Ferry.

At the time of the Harpers Ferry incident, Smith and Brown had been friends and collaborators in the anti-slavery movement for more than a decade. Smith was even a member of the Secret Committee of Six, which was a group of six wealthy and powerful men who financially supported John Brown's anti-slavery tactics. Membership in the committee was kept secret in part because Brown's tactics were growing increasingly radical. After more than two decades of dedication to the abolitionist cause, Brown became increasingly convinced that peaceful and non-violent methods of ending slavery were ineffective. He decided that more drastic tactics were required.

Brown's plan for Harpers Ferry involved capturing a federal armory and using the captured guns and ammunition to lead a massive slave rebellion throughout the South. It is not known for certain whether Smith and the other members of the Secret Committee of Six were fully aware of Brown's plan, but they did meet with Brown several times in the months leading up to the incident, and their financial support of Brown undoubtedly aided his efforts. It is generally thought that the members of the Six, including Smith, were ambivalent about or actually against Brown's suggested use of violence as a means to end slavery.

New York Lunatic Asylum at Utica

The Harpers Ferry incident turned out to be a total disaster. Brown and 21 other men, including five black men, attempted to rob the armory at Harpers Ferry on the morning of October 16th, 1859. They managed to capture several buildings before a freed black man not associated with the plot was killed by Brown's gunfire, and the shots alerted local residents to the incident. Brown and his fellow raiders were soon surrounded, disarmed, and arrested. Brown was eventually tried and hung as a traitor. The incident was seen by many as a demonstration of the increasingly volatile nature of the relationship between those in favor of slavery and those against it. Many historians consider the raid at Harpers Ferry as a major impetus to the Civil War.

After the incident, Senator Jefferson Davis attempted to have Smith tried and hanged like John Brown, but was ultimately not successful in this attempt. Smith later claimed that he did not know about Brown's plans for a violent raid leading to a slave uprising. He claimed he thought Brown simply wanted access to weapons in order to provide runaway slaves with a means for defending themselves when necessary. It was in the aftermath of the raid that Smith became a patient at the New York State Lunatic Asylum in Utica.

Smith claimed to have had a mental breakdown sparked by the stressful days and weeks following the Harpers Ferry incident. Whether or not Smith knew the details of Brown's plan and was complicit in it, the negative attention and scrutiny the incident drew to Smith would certainly have been cause for stress and anxiety. The New York State Lunatic Asylum would have provided him with a peaceful and quiet refuge for regaining his emotional strength and calming his nerves. On the other hand, some contemporaries of Smith as well as modern-day historians believe he was feigning his mental breakdown as a way to escape arrest and possible hanging. There was certainly ample evidence linking Smith to the incident, including a personal check from Smith to Brown found in Brown's pocket at the time of his arrest. No consensus has ever been reached on this, as Smith would have had good reasons for feigning his mental illness, but equally good reasons for genuinely suffering from it. (45)

The Utica Crib

Unfortunately, not all treatment methods performed at the New York State Lunatic Asylum seem quite so humane or reasonable in hindsight. During his time at the Utica asylum, Dr. Brigham invented the soon to become notorious "Utica crib method". This invention was actually a modification of an existing "restraint bed" that Dr. Brigham encountered at a facility in France. He modified the restraint bed to be more humane and his version became known as the "Utica crib," which was soon in use at many of the mental institutions rapidly being built throughout the country.

The crib in question was an adult-sized wooden bed modeled after a baby's crib. The crib had a top that closed down over the patient and could be locked. The crib was made from open wooden slats in order to allow air flow, and the bottom of the crib was lined with straw to provide some softness and comfort. The crib could also be suspended on chains and rocked to soothe an especially distraught patient. Generally, only violent or agitated patients who were thought to be badly in need of rest, and who refused to remain in their own beds, were placed in the crib.

The Utica crib came to be widely criticized and eventually fell out of favor. It was especially unpopular among patients at the New York State Lunatic Asylum, whom understandably did not enjoy the feeling of extreme confinement and entrapment created by the crib. Not everyone was critical, however, with at least one Utica patient insisting that the crib allowed him to experience deeply therapeutic rest, beneficial for "all crazy fellows as

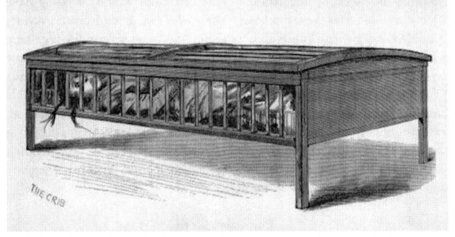

The Utica Crib, named after the site of its invention, was heavily used during the 19th-century to confine and control patients. Although harshly criticized, some found it had important therapeutic value.

I, whose spirit is willing, but whose flesh is weak," (Journal of Insanity, October 1864).

While the Utica crib might seem horrifyingly inhumane and barbaric today, it is important to view its use within the appropriate context. At the time that Dr. Brigham created this form of therapy; residential mental institutions were still a new and innovative phenomenon. At the time, the mentally ill were routinely confined and locked away, not only with locks on the doors of the attics or dark basements where they were kept, but also by being chained to the wall or the floor. Dr. Brigham considered such confinement to be incredibly inhumane and of no benefit to the patient. (46)

His New York State Lunatic Asylum did not feature heavy padlocked doors or barred windows. To the contrary, the asylum was a wide open space allowing most patients a lot of freedom of movement. He conceived of the Utica crib not as a medieval torture device, but rather as the most humane alternative he could come up with for those severely agitated patients who required restraint in order to be subdued. The crib also served as a safety measure intended to prevent certain patients from harming either themselves or others, and in fact was credited with saving the life of at least one suicidal female patient in Utica. While it's easy to see the Utica crib as a nightmarish tool of entrapment, it was intended to provide severely upset patients with a safe and comfortable place to achieve rest.

The Fate of the New York State Lunatic Asylum

The New York State Lunatic Asylum was continually in use for more than a century, not closing until the 1970's. At various times it was known as the Utica Lunatic Asylum, Utica State Hospital, and the Utica Psychiatric Center. Locally, the building has long been referred to as Old Main. By the 1970's many residential mental asylums across the U.S. began to close due to further changes in the field of psychiatry. With the increasing popularity of prescribed pharmaceutical medication for various mental illnesses, many symptoms of mental illness could be kept under control on an out-patient basis.

Large, grand mental health facilities like the asylum in Utica were also quite expensive to maintain and operate. Most states chose to slow public funding for mental institutions, leaving only smaller residential facilities for more extremely mentally ill patients. The closing of the New York State Lunatic Asylum in 1978 was typical for institutions of its type. Since its closing, the building itself has stood mostly unoccupied and has fallen into disrepair. It became a National Historic Landmark in 1989. The building does remain, however, of both architectural and historic interest to many. The New York State Office of Mental Health renovated a small portion of the first floor in 2004, and has since used it as a Records Archive and Repository. Though various uses for the rest of the building have been proposed over the years, funds have not been forthcoming, and the beautiful old building that was once the site of so much hope and progress remains unoccupied and neglected. (47)

Chapter 9

New York Asylum for Idiots at Syracuse

The Syracuse State School was a residential facility located in Syracuse, New York for mentally disabled children and adults. Founded in 1851, its first director was Hervey B. Wilbur. Wilbur stated in his first annual report, "The Idiot Institution is more properly a school than an asylum. No inmates are received beyond the age at which instruction is not usually available, nor any who do not seem likely to profit by it".

Wilbur's report also points out that "these idiots were young, and that they could be taught. They were free of the habits of older idiots, and were more flexible, and susceptible to development. There was more of a chance to correct their physical defects or infirmities through diet or medicine. They were generally happy, affectionate, obedient, and easily amused".

Out of the initial twenty-five students in the asylum, twelve could not speak. Out of the twelve that couldn't speak, six did not understand language at all. Of the students who were not "dumb", three of them spoke a few words, but indistinctly. Two others didn't say a word until they were nine years old and even then indistinctly and only a few words. Seven of the students walked imperfectly, three had a partial paralysis, eleven had seizures, eight drooled, and seven were incontinent. Several of the students had to be watched constantly because of health issues related to cleanliness, and five of the students were "irritable." Most were unable to dress or undress themselves, and only four students could feed themselves. None of the students could read, write or distinguish colors by name.

In 1855 the facility moved to a new building in Syracuse where it was known as the New York Asylum for Idiots or the State Idiot Asylum. Over the next hundred years the institution went through several name changes, including the Syracuse State Institution for Feeble-Minded Children, the Syracuse State School for Mental Defectives, and finally the Syracuse State School in 1927. The school was closed in 1973 and the building was torn down in 1988. (48)

From the Archives of the Syracuse Asylum

In 2008, Syracuse University purchased a remarkable collection now housed in their Special Collections Department called, The James Thornton Correspondence. These letters are not written by James Thornton (also called "Jamie" and "Jimmy") but rather consist of correspondence between various staff members including the director of the asylum Dr. Hervey B.Wilbur to James Thornton's mother. Unfortunately her letters are not included in the collection but we can infer some of her concerns and thoughts judging from the response letters from the staff. There are a total of 23 letters in the collection.

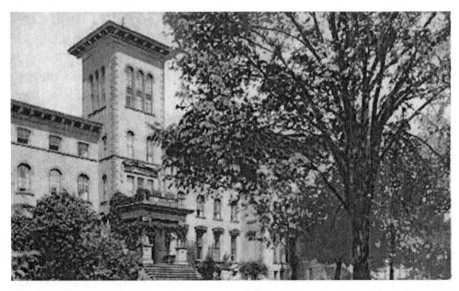

The New York Asylum for Idiots was founded in Syracuse in 1851. Over the next hundred years the institution went through several name changes eventually becoming known as the Syracuse State School.

New York Asylum for Idiots at Syracuse

The James Thornton Correspondence

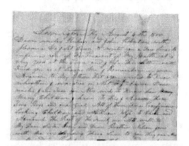

The James Thornton Correspondence consists of letters written by the Director, Hervey B. Wilbur and other staff members to the mother of James (Jimmy) Thornton, described only as a "little boy" who was admitted to the asylum in 1855.

What we know from the letters is that Jimmy Thornton was probably around seven years old when he entered the asylum at Syracuse in September, 1855. We also know from the letters that he would have been one of the very first pupils in the new building at Syracuse after the asylum moved from Albany in 1854. We know Dr. R. H. Gray of Cinncinatus, New York most likely wrote the letter of application for Jimmy's admittance, as the first letter in the collection is written to Dr. Gray from Dr. Wilbur requesting the name and address of the mother of "the little boy from Cinncinatus." Jimmy's mother was Mrs. Mary Thornton, also from Cinncinatus, who became Mrs. Mary Whead when she remarried in 1859 and thus moved further away from the asylum to Caton, New York. We know that this move and her remarriage must have somehow influenced her relationship with her son and her relationship to the asylum, as we can observe a marked change in circumstances around 1859 which corresponds to Mrs. Thornton's remarriage and her request, for various possible reasons, for Jimmy not to return for a visit home. From the letters, we also know that Jimmy Thornton was deaf, did not speak, knew sign language, and read and wrote in English. We know he most likely attended the school as a state-funded pupil, which indicates that his mother was too poor to pay for his special schooling. Even after her remarriage in 1859, it appears that Jimmy continued on as a state-funded pupil (rather than the family paying for his institutionalization) since there is no indication in the letters that his status changed. We cannot be completely certain of Mrs. Thornton's financial status before or after her second marriage nor can we be sure of the ways in which her remarriage and re-location further away from the asylum-school affected her relationship with Jimmy and with the asylum's administration. We do know that there is none of Jimmy's writings left, even though he is said to have been able to write a "good copy." While Jimmy was given reasonable access to basic bi-lingual literacy education, through his learning to read and write English and American Sign Language, it is significant that in the historical record he remains silent—but certainly, not absent.

What follows is an extraordinary series of letters which perhaps give us a unique insight into the world of an, 'asylum for idiots'. (49)

The Little Boy from Cinncinatus

The very first letter of the correspondence, dated September 7, 1855, is from Superintendent Wilbur to Dr. Gray, the authorizing physician from the town in which the Thornton's lived. The letter signals an initial intent of reassurance and consolation, though brief, that points to the potentiality of the asylum's new acquisition, referred to anonymously as "the little boy from Cinncinatus."

Dr. Wilbur begins his letter to Dr. Gray reassuring him that the boy has arrived and is well:

Dear Sir,
The little boy from Cincinnatus is very well and quite at home and contented with us. I think that he will make a very good pupil. If you will, please to write to me giving the name and P.O. address of the mother—I will write to her occasionally of her child's welfare.
Yours Truly
H.B. Wilbur (Letter One, Sept. 7, 1855)

Some weeks later, Matron Mrs. E.F. Mulford, attempts to console Mrs. Thornton with a brief description of Jimmy's experience. The letter goes as follows:

I hope you will hear [through the intermediary] a favorable account of your boy's progress and feel satisfied that he remembers you for really I was quite surprised to see him show so much emotion—he actually shed tears. But this gentleman who is the bearer of this will tell you all.
From The Matron Mrs. E.F. Mulford (Letter Two, undated).

New York Asylum for Idiots at Syracuse

In letter three, Wilbur writes six months into Jimmy's stay:

He will be very glad to see you—though for the present, a visit from you might make him homesick again. (Letter Three, Oct. 8, 1855)

Mrs. Thornton wrote back to Wilbur quite quickly after his letter of rebuke, and in her letter back to him she must have expressed her displeasure. The entirety of Wilbur's response comes two weeks after Mrs. Thornton could have requested a visit, indicating that the issue over visitation constituted the most intensive period of correspondence (the most number of letters back and forth in the shortest timeframe). The letter goes as follows:

Dear Madam,
I have but little time to write letters and many letters to write, so that I have to write short letters to all the friends of my pupils. Your little boy is very happy here now. He is very desirous of learning and will in time make an excellent pupil. He is a favorite with all, as I think, I wrote you before.
Yours truly H.B. Wilbur (Letter Four, October 22, 1855)

Superintendent Wilbur reassures Mrs. Thornton a year into Jimmy's schooling:

Your little boy continues well—he is perfectly happy in his new home and getting on nicely in school matters. He is an affectionate little fellow and all the teachers and attendants are quite attracted to him. (Letter Five, Nov. 20, 1855)

Wilbur's assistant H.H. Saville goes on to console the family in another letter a year later. As Saville tells us, Wilbur does not have enough time to write to all the families, so Saville writes for him:

Your little boy is perfectly well and very well supplied with clothes. He appears perfectly contented and his teachers like him very much. Indeed he is a favorite with everybody in the Asylum. I hope you feel quite easy about him for he seems healthy and he is much more in the way of improvement here than could possibly be at home.
Yours Truly, H.H. Saville for Dr. H.B. Wilbur. (Letter Seven, Sept. 1, 1856)

In letter nine, the Matron Mulford writes:

He came in our dining room and took dinner with the family on Sunday noon. He was somewhat nervous but still enjoyed it very much. He is a sweet affectionate child and a general favorite. We made him understand that he with the other children are to have a fine time Christmas—we always devote our undivided attention to their amusement on that day and the Dr. will make them all some little present—Jamie has sufficient clothing for the winter—do not give yourself the least [illegible] for my assistant takes the best care of him. He always kisses me a sweet goodnight.
Yours reply E.F. Mulford (Letter Nine, Dec. 15, 1856)

Perhaps she is more detailed than Saville or Wilbur because Mulford is engaged in the everyday routine of the asylum. Mulford also apologizes as Saville did, in the following letter, for Wilbur being absent as the letter-writer.

Again the Dr. has availed himself of my services in the letter writing department. I can only say that your boy is well, happy, and doing well in school...I have many letters to write and must hasten from one to another.
Briefly but sincerely yours E.F. Mulford (Letter Ten, Jan. 21, 1857)

In letter eleven, she writes:

He is a darling boy and he improves so much in school—is so easily managed. He can put up a great many words on the letter board and read almost any word on the blackboard. He is perfectly well and enjoys himself-We have more than one hundred pupils and but one case of sickness
Yours in haste E.F. Mulford (Letter 11, March 25, 1857)

L. Hutchinson's letters (Jimmy's teacher) demonstrate that she observed Jimmy first-hand and worked with him daily. Her first letter is brief (Letter 13), essentially attesting that he is a good pupil, is well, and is in good health. Her following letters (Letters 14 & 15) offer more educational information. Hutchinson writes:

New York Asylum for Idiots at Syracuse

He seems very much delighted with any exercise and perhaps it would be gratifying to you to know that. I consider him one of the best pupils under my charge. He can write anything with a copy before him and a great many words and sentences without [copy]. He is also learning to read but slowly of course because you know he is deaf and dumb and obliged to be taught wholly by signs.
Yours Respectfully,
L. Hutchinson (Letter 14, March 3, 1858)

In the letter dated July, 10, 1859, Harriet Wilbur, Superintendent Wilbur's wife, attempts to persuade Mrs. Whead (her new, married name) to send for her son so Jimmy would not have to stay at the asylum through summer vacation (Letter 16, July 15, 1859). Mrs. Wilbur writes:

The annual vacation of the Asylum commences on the Monday of next July 18th instant. Your son is very desirous of going home and Dr. Wilbur wishes me to say that he wishes it also. You will please reply to this immediately [her underline] and state when you will come or send for him.

This constitutes the second major shift in the correspondence (again, focused on the issue of visitation) because now Jimmy's wishes are not only voiced but are also attempted to be carried out ("Your son is very desirous of going home"). But, Mrs. Whead must have responded by requesting that Jimmy stay on at the asylum through the summer of 1859—at which point Mrs. Wilbur responds:

Dr. Wilbur wishes me to say in reply to the letter of yours of date of July 25, that your son can remain through the vacation. He is very well. (Letter 17, Aug. 1, 1859)

Wilbur writes:

Mrs. Whead, Dear Madam
Should you like to have your son Jimmy come home if I would send him to Elmira without expense to you? Would you meet him there and like him home, if I would write you? It would do him much good to go home.
Yours Truly H.B. Wilbur (Letter 18, July 1861)

From a future correspondence we learn that, in fact, James went home to visit his mother in the summer of 1861.

Six months after James Thornton left the asylum, in January of 1862, he still had not returned to Syracuse. Four years later still Jimmy had not returned and no word from Mrs. Whead. On January 8, 1866, Dr. Wilbur communicates in his final letter what seems an almost desperate situation. This salient moment demonstrates how dynamics and lines of arguments shifted once the pupil left. It is Wilbur who is pleading for information—Wilbur himself takes time to write:

Is [Jimmy] still living? What is his state of health? How has he grown? What does he do and how does he amuse himself? Does he ever speak of his life here? We were talking about him the other day, and I cannot resist the desire to hear from him once more. Please write me about him…What has become of Jimmy Thornton, as we used to call him?
…I remain yours truly, H.B. Wilbur (Letter 19, Jan. 1866)

And, thus, we are left contemplating the same question: what has become of Jimmy Thornton? Unfortunately, we will never know. (50)

Chapter 10
New York State Inebriate Asylum at Binghamton

The New York State Inebriate Hospital was founded in 1858 in Binghamton, New York. Like many of the mental institutions built in the United States during the mid-19th century, the Inebriate Hospital was designed as an elegantly imposing Gothic revival building, surrounded by grounds and farmland belonging to the hospital.

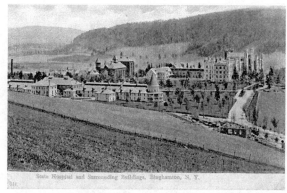

The New York State Inebriate Asylum in Binghamton, New York was founded in 1858. It was the first of its kind established in the world.

The hospital was designed by the well-known and prolific architect Isaac G. Perry. Unlike many of its contemporary institutions, the Inebriate Hospital was initially intended as a hospital for the treatment of alcoholics, only transitioning to a residential mental health institution at a later date. It was the first institution of its kind founded anywhere in the world.

In many ways the history of the treatment of alcoholics mirrors that of the treatment of the mentally ill. At the time that the New York State Inebriate Hospital was founded by Dr. J. Edward Turner, alcoholics were mostly seen by society as a nuisance and an embarrassment, rather than people with a sickness that could be treated. While Dorothea Dix was campaigning for reform in the treatment of the mentally ill, arguing that many of them would be cured through a humane combination of medical and moral therapy, Turner was arguing the same for the chronically inebriate. The New York State Inebriate Hospital was founded with the belief that alcoholism, at the time usually referred to as "dipsomania," could be treated as "a disease, requiring . . . for its cure, medical and moral treatment" (Castle on a Hill). (51)

Dr. J. Edward Turner

Dr. J. Edward Turner was a medical doctor and reformer whose personal experiences helped contribute to his interest in reform of the way alcoholism was treated. Early in his medical career, Dr. Turner treated his own uncle for symptoms of alcoholism. Rather than treat his uncle as an annoying or embarrassing pest, as was the norm at the time, Dr. Turner treated his uncle as though he had an illness which could be treated through lack of access to alcohol, and an emphasis on nutritious food, physical exercise, and moral teachings.

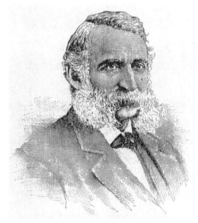

Dr. J. Edward Turner (1822-1889) an institutional reformer who believed alcoholism was a disease and required treatment. His approach would be met with fierce opposition.

The treatment of his uncle must have been at least fairly successful because this experience led to Dr. Turner's interest in treating alcoholism on a larger scale in a residential setting, in a similar manner to the way the mentally ill were beginning to be treated. Dr. Turner founded the New York State Inebriate Hospital, the first hospital in the world dedicated to the treatment of alcohol addiction, and served as its first superintendent. Dr. Turner created and operated the asylum under the, at the time, revolutionary theory that "the inebriate, without an asylum, perils his own life by his own hand, jeopardizes the lives of others, and dies the most painful death" (Castle on the Hill). The asylum under Dr. Turner's watch was dedicated to counteracting and preventing these tragedies from occurring. As such, patients were treated almost more like students at a benign boarding school than inmates. (52)

Transition to Insane Asylum and Later Years

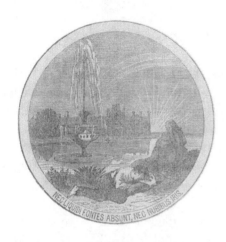

In 1867 asylum founder, Dr. Turner resigns. By 1872 the asylum reached its highest population of 334 patients. In 1879 Governor Lucious Robinson declares the inebriate asylum a failure and recommends conversion to an asylum for the chronically insane.

While the inebriate asylum in Binghamton was founded with the best of intentions, unfortunately, by 1879 it was considered wildly unsuccessful, even being officially declared "a complete failure" by the governor of New York. It is unclear exactly what caused the asylum to fail, but what is known is that the patient population steadily declined over time, and by 1878 only 38 patients remained compared to 334 in 1872. The inebriate asylum was closed in 1879, but rather than abandon the facility altogether, an insane asylum was opened in the same building in 1881 as the Binghamton Asylum for the Chronic Insane.

As an insane asylum, the facility was considered significantly more successful, housing as many as 600 patients at one point in its history. The Binghamton Asylum for the Chronic Insane was the site of many firsts in mental health, including many mental health treatment methods that have since fallen out of favor but were considered very innovative at the time. For example, the first electro-shock therapy was performed at the Binghamton Asylum for the Chronic Insane in 1942, followed by the first lobotomy in 1946. Then in 1955 the asylum in Binghamton became the first hospital in the country to prescribe medication for the treatment of mental illness.

The Binghamton Asylum for the Chronic Insane was renamed the probably less stigmatic Binghamton State Hospital in 1890, and then again renamed the Binghamton Psychiatric Center in 1974. After years of dwindling use, the building was officially closed in 1993 and has long sat in abandoned decay. As of 2008, however, the state government of New York has begun dedicating a large amount of money and resources to its renovation, with the intention of turning it into a campus for the SUNY Upstate Medical University.(53)

Wet Packing

One of the strangest treatment practices at the Binghamton asylum was what was known as wet packing, also known as hydrotherapy. This practice was intended to sedate and restrain agitated patients, in a similar manner to the Utica crib or the use of straightjackets, and like those practices it met with mixed results and controversy. Unlike the Utica crib or the use of straightjackets, wet packing was intended to be more bracing and invigorating than comforting. It was also said to be used as punishment, rather than treatment, for certain patients who "acted up."

In wet packing, a table would be placed in the middle of the room, and then covered with a pile of ten blankets. On top of the ten blankets would be placed an additional ten bed sheets, which had been dunked in ice water and then rung out. The patient would then strip out of their clothes and lie on top of the table, over the blankets and the cold, wet sheets. They would then be "packed in" and wrapped like a mummy in the layers of blankets and sheets. Next, they would be rolled off the table onto the floor and tied down. The unfortunate patients treated in this manner would remain "wet packed" for six hours, with only their feet and hands free from the packing. This practice continued at the Binghamton asylum until the late 1950's, until a young patient named Gerald died while being wet packed, supposedly from a brain aneurism brought on by his violently struggling against his blanket and sheet restraints. (54)

Paranormal Activity at the New York State Inebriate Asylum

Like many old, abandoned insane asylums, the asylum in Binghamton is considered by many to be the site of paranormal and ghost activity. In 2003, the Paranormal and Ghosts Society performed a study at the old asylum, and declared that both the building and surrounding grounds were certifiably haunted. The paranormal investigators claimed that the grounds were actually the site of more paranormal activity than the buildings themselves, and claim to have photographed several ghosts on the grounds. These ghosts were presumed to be former patients, who would have worked on the grounds as well as had recreational time there as part of their treatment. The paranormal investigators admit they had limited time to explore the facility and grounds, so it is possible that with more time they may have detected more paranormal activity within the buildings themselves. Even though, like most mid-19th century mental facilities, the New York State Inebriate Hospital was founded with altruistic and kind intentions, it was no doubt the site of much pain and turmoil. If there is in fact such a thing as ghosts, there's probably no more likely place for them to be than a long-abandoned inebriate and mental asylum, where for more than a hundred years various alcoholics, drug addicts, and mentally ill were housed, often against their will and in some cases treated in way now considered excessively inhumane. (55)

Chapter 11
Willard Asylum for the Insane

It has been reported that her name was Mary Rote. She arrived by steamboat at Ovid Landing on Seneca Lake, about 65 miles southeast of Rochester, New York. Described as "deformed and demented," she was chained at the wrists and transported by armed guards to the Willard Asylum for the Chronic Insane. She was to be their first patient. The year was 1869. (56)

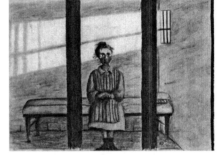

Mary Rote (B.?-D.?) Willard's first patient. Dropped off by steamboat in shackles. Spent the previous ten years often naked and chained to a wall.

Mary's journey had been a long time coming. In truth, it had begun decades earlier when another woman, Dorothea Lynda Dix of Massachusetts, made her first assault on the New York State Legislature to reform the poorhouses, almshouses, asylums, and jails where the state's "lunatics" were kept. Dix spent her whole adult life lobbying governors, legislatures, the United States Congress, even foreign governments, to improve the living conditions of the insane and destitute who were housed under the most horrific conditions wherever they were found throughout the "civilized world." She is said to have single-handedly reformed the systems of asylum in at least eighteen states over the course of her career as a social activist. (See Chapter One for Dix bio.)

Willard Asylum for the Insane

The Chronically Insane

In 1864, under pressure from Dix, the New York State Legislature tasked the state's Surgeon General, Dr. Sylvester D. Willard, to investigate conditions within these "institutions" and to come back with recommendations. Several months later, Willard reported that in 55 New York counties, not including New York City, there were 1355 individuals, adjudged to be "chronically insane," living in "deplorable" conditions. In response to the report, Governor Reuben Fenton signed a bill drawn up by Dr. Willard and other M.D.s, and spearheaded through the legislature by Senator Charles Folger of Geneva, authorizing the establishment of the State Asylum for the Chronic Insane. Shortly thereafter, Dr. Willard passed away and both the bill and the institution it would establish were named for him.

Signed into law on April 8, 1865, just six days before President Lincoln's assassination, the Willard bill provided for the transfer of all persons residing in county poorhouses throughout the state to a new facility to be erected on the site of the abandoned Ovid Agricultural College in Ovid, New York. Though there were some existing buildings on the site, a "modern" facility would soon be under construction. Thus began the mass warehousing of the mentally ill in New York State, and the first "treatment" of New York's mentally ill population. (57)

Insane Persons

From colonial times, the care of "insane persons" in New York and most other states had been a local function. Each county operated a poorhouse, or almshouse where "dependent persons" were housed. These included the homeless, the aged, the crippled, drunks, epileptics, beggars, the feebleminded, and the mad. Some of these poorhouses were nothing more than county jails. These facilities provided custody and shelter, but "treatment" was not part of the equation. The inhabitants of these "shelters" were collectively categorized as the "pauper lunatic class" or the "chronic insane." Whether or not those were appropriate descriptions of those who entered, they were generally accurate for any who remained for even short periods of incarceration . . . which brings us back to Mary Rote. The first patient to arrive at Willard for treatment, Mary had been chained for 10 years without a bed and without clothing in a cell in the Columbia County almshouse. Later that day, three more patients, all male, arrived at the dock, in irons--one in what has been described as a "chicken crate," 3 1/2 feet square. Many of the early patients at Willard had been considered "difficult" and were "quieted" by regular flogging, dousing and hanging by the thumbs in the almshouses.

By 1869, a "modern" asylum building had been constructed at Willard. Like the Eastern and Great Meadow prisons, the asylum was built on the approved institutional design of the day--a three-story center structure for administration with long wings radiating from either side for patient housing, males in one wing and females in the other. Within a few months of opening, admissions outstripped the building's 250-bed capacity, and the former college building, high on the hill overlooking the lake, was renovated as housing for higher-functioning patients.

By the end of the first year, with the census approaching 700, Willard began to construct "detached buildings" away from the main building. The detached buildings housed working patients and their attendants. Willard was growing rapidly.

By 1877, with more than 1,500 patients, it was the largest asylum in the United States. By 1890, when the name was changed to Willard State Hospital and its function enlarged to include acute as well as chronic patients, Willard had become a small city, with over 70 buildings and 2000 patients.

During its first 20 years of operation, the "treatment" that took place within its fences and walls is largely a matter of speculation based on anecdotal evidence, archeological findings, a few hand-written first-hand accounts from staff and their families, and extrapolated knowledge of generalized mental health practices of this bygone era. Though many records do exist in various archives of the state, it seems that

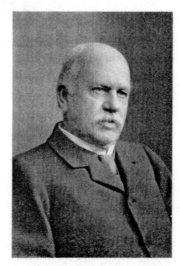

JOHN B. CHAPIN, M.D., LL.D.

Dr. John B. Chapin (1829-1918) Willard's first superintendent. From his obituary; "Formed on the good old plan, a true and brave and downright honest man. Loathing pretense, he did with cheerful will, what others talked off, while their hands were still".

doctor-patient confidentiality is protected under law well beyond the lifetimes of doctors or patients. Yet, other kinds of investigations have pieced together a reasonable portrait of Willard over the course of its lifetime. (58)

The first Medical Superintendent at Willard was Dr. John B. Chapin who had previously worked with mentally ill patients in Utica, New York. Chapin compiled a scrapbook, now in the Cornell University Library, containing newspaper articles pertaining to Willard. One such article, appearing in the New York Times on March 21, 1872, tells of a young woman who had been brought to Willard after years of being chained by the ankle to the floor in a room 5-feet square, in a poorhouse, in a nearby county because she was disturbed and destructive. According to Chapin who was quoted in the article, the woman had been flogged with a whip and a strap for years by the local superintendent who told Chapin that "pulling" her--hanging her by her thumbs--had been the only effective treatment. The article went on to say that the reporter who visited Willard and interviewed Chapin saw patients sitting quietly in their wards, clean and decently dressed. (59)

Therapy

Over the years, many forms of treatment were used at Willard. In the 1890s, it was believed that most mental illness was due to Syphilis. At Willard, treatment for Syphilis-induced mental illness consisted primarily of giving patients Thyroid Extract. Desiccated thyroid glands from pigs and cows were administered to patients in varying dosages. Not a single success was reported. Arsenic and Malaria was also tried and according to some reports from that period, some patients showed improvement. Another form of treatment used during the first decades of Willard's operation was Insulin Coma Therapy. This was a commonly used Psychiatric treatment in which patients were repeatedly injected with large doses of insulin order to produce daily comas over several weeks. The effectiveness of this therapy was reported as "mixed." The drug Metrazol was also used for a period of time. Also known as Pentetrazol, it is a circulatory and respiratory stimulant which in high doses causes convulsions. Never proven to be effective, the side-effects such as seizures were often more destructive than helpful.

Others therapies used at Willard included Electro-shock Therapy, Hydrotherapy, Occupational Therapy, Music Therapy, and Physiotherapy.

The effectiveness of these treatments was summed up in a historical document prepared by a Dr. Kiel in 1948. "The outstanding treatment is the kindly and considerate care given by the staff and employees and the food preparation and service, all of these activities are simply preliminary to basis Psychotherapy. They tend to show the patient who has frequently been neglected or rejected that people in the hospital are interested in his welfare and thereby restore him to a frame of mind where he is willing and able to discuss his problems with a Psychiatrist and receive suggestions and advice or more tangible assistance as needed."

In a recent Internet blog posting, authored by a woman who identified herself only as Eileen, she speaks of a visit she made to Willard, and of a document she had located that described the early days of the asylum's operation. Authored by Dr. Robert E. Doran, the document suggests the treatments given during the early years at Willard were much less sinister. The early years of treatment were labeled as "moral treatment" or "custodial care", and as Dr. Doran explained, "Patients were treated with kindness, given good but not fancy food, given clothes, exercised, and protected from the outside world." Doran goes on to write that in 1883, there were 801 patients willing and able to work. He does, however, go on to suggest that such able-bodied workers were often kept at Willard indefinitely because their services were needed. (60)

"I grew up not far from Willard," writes another blogger. "The asylum was open, but only whispered about. I grew up hearing the horror stories about the crazies, the straight-jackets and the lobotomies. It was said, 'Once you went to Willard, you never came out.' " (61)

The Grave Digger Lawrence

The foregoing is an assertion that is supported, in no small measure, by the over 5700 unmarked graves in the Willard Asylum Cemetery.

According to Jennifer Burke, writing in the July 25, 2011 edition of the Catholic Courier, "In 1918 an Austrian immigrant named Lawrence arrived at Willard Asylum, the state mental hospital on the shores of Seneca Lake that would become his home for the next 50 years. A veteran of the Royal Austrian Army, this man was no stranger to mental institutions. He'd previously spent time in mental hospitals in Germany and Long Island, where he reportedly sang, shouted, and whistled boisterously and sometimes claimed to hear the voice of God and see angels.

Lawrence was a hard worker and became the hospital's unpaid gravedigger in 1937. Over the course of the previous three decades he dug hundreds of graves in Willard Cemetery and even obtained permission to live in a small shack on the cemetery grounds in the warmer months. In 1968 he died at the age of 90, and became one of the permanent residents of the cemetery he'd toiled in for 30 years.

Colleen Spellecy, a member of St. Mary Parish in Waterloo, couldn't stop thinking about Lawrence after she read his story in *The Lives They Left Behind: Suitcases From a State Hospital Attic*. The 2008 book by Darby Penney and Peter Stasny details the lives of 10 Willard residents whose belongings were among those found in an attic on the hospital grounds after the facility closed in 1995. The authors did not disclose Willard residents' last names because of privacy concerns.

Spellecy was troubled when she learned that Lawrence and most of the 5,775 others resting in Willard Cemetery do not have grave markers bearing their names.

"That really bothered me, that he dug over 900 graves and no one knows where he's buried," Spellecy said.

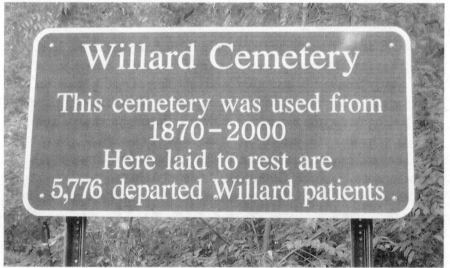

When the State closed the Willard Psychiatric Center in 1995, it was discovered that 5700 patients were buried there, often in unmarked graves.

The graves of most Willard residents were marked with stones bearing numbers, rather than names, but many of those original markers have since been moved, she added. Spellecy was appalled at the cemetery's unkempt condition the first time she visited, and its condition hasn't improved, she said. Many of the markers that were moved were replaced with corresponding numbers on concrete-filled pipes dug into the ground. These newer markers are hard to find, however, because the cemetery is mowed no more than twice a year.

Spellecy believes the state of the cemetery and its unnamed graves is an insult to the dignity of the people who are buried there. Proper and respectful burial of the dead is important in both Christian and Jewish traditions, but that respect is lacking in Willard Cemetery, which has special sections for Catholics, Jews, Protestants and even Civil War veterans. The graves of the Civil War veterans are the only ones marked by headstones labeled with names. (62)

"The rest remain faceless, they remain nameless, and their relatives can't even go visit them because they don't know where they are," Spellecy said. Such is the following story of Lucy Ann Lobdell, but unlike those who occupy one of Willard's unmarked graves, she was to suffer an even more terrible fate.

The Female Hunter of Delaware County

Born in 1829 to a working-class family in upstate-New York, Lucy Ann Lobdell was not your average girl. Donning her brother's clothes, she worked on the family farm and in her father's saw mill, demonstrating marksmanship skills that earned her the nickname "The Female Hunter of Delaware County". After leaving home, she moved to the frontier, married a woman, and lived for sixty years as a man named "Joe". Because of nineteenth-century social restrictions and gender expectations, Lobdell endured forced marriage, arrest, and incarceration in the Willard Insane Asylum. Although twentieth-century scholars have labeled her a lesbian, stories about Lucy and Joe, and Lobdell's own writings reveal that she was actually transgendered.

Even after being incarcerated in Willard, Lobdell continued to dress in male attire and declared herself to be a man, giving her name as Joseph Lobdell, a Methodist minister. When Lucy/Joe was interviewed by psychiatrist, Dr. Wise at Willard, Dr. Wise stated that his patient was lucid, clear, coherent, not confused, not erratic, and able to relate vivid recollections of 'her/his' life. Incredibly though, Dr. Wise concluded that his patient was delusional and stated that "everyone knows sex without a penis is impossible", which Lucy of course did not have.

As the result Lucy would spend the last 33 years of her life incarcerated at Willard for insisting she was a man and would die in 1912. But it was when she was first admitted to Willard in 1879, that Marie, Lucy's 'wife', had been told that Lucy was dead! Marie, not considered by society as the legal wife of Lucy, subsequently had her farm confiscated by the county as well as losing Lucy's pension. In 1878, Lucy's brother John helped her receive 15 years of back widows pension she was entitled to because a man who she

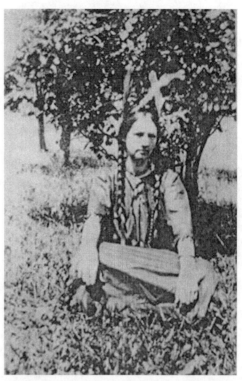

Lucy Ann Lobdell (1829-1912) today she would probably be thought of as a lesbian or transgendered. Admitted to Willard in 1880 because of her sexual orientation, she would spend the last 33 years of her life incarcerated in mental institutions.

had been forced to marry years earlier, had been killed in the Civil War. Marie tried to live in the woods on the survival skills she had learned from Lucy, but she was not successful. She eventually became beloved by her community near Honesdale, PA, and the town's people would allow her to stay in their barns and homes. Marie finally made her way back to her childhood home of Whitman, MA. She worked in a factory until she died in 1890. (63)

***

While the stories of those confined to Willard may never be fully told, efforts are underway today to open the asylum's records to the public and interested families. Though it is unlikely that the remains of the former residents who still inhabit the Willard grounds will ever be ascertained, we do know that among them is Lawrence the grave digger, Willard's first patient, Mary Rote and The Female Hunter of Delaware County.

May God have mercy on their souls.

Chapter 12
Hudson River Hospital
for the Insane

The place is downright spooky. Stephen King spooky. Beyond Stephen King spooky. More like Edgar Allen Poe meets Bram Stoker spooky.

Sitting on a hill overlooking the Hudson River, spellbinding for its High Victorian Gothic architecture, what once was the Hudson River Asylum for the Insane is now best described as a Hollywood set-piece for amateur

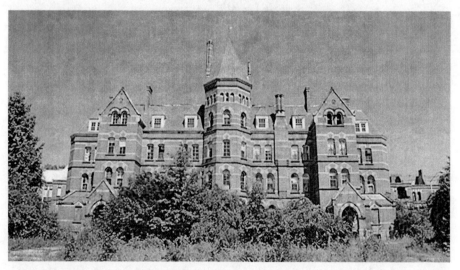

The Hudson River State Hospital opened in 1871. The campus is notable for its main building, due to the "Kirkbride" design. The institution has been designated a National Historic Landmark.

videographers, paranormal investigators, and connoisseurs of the creepy. It attracts rabid mobs of architecture buffs, historians, archeologists, sociologists, photographers, and haunted house enthusiasts. In Poughkeepsie, New York, it is the place to be on Halloween.

The Internet is filled with photographs of its buildings and grounds, dating back to its construction in the 1870s, '80s, and '90s. (It took that long to build.) Part of the "Renaissance" in the care and treatment of the mentally ill in New York, it was funded and operated by the State and it's as famous for its exorbitant price-tag (over $1 million) as it is for the horror stories that justify its highly regarded spookiness.

"The beauty of the decay was unbelievable . . ." writes a blogger on the popular website, forbiddenplaces.net after visiting the hospital which sits on hundreds of acres of tangled weeds and bushes. "It is said that screams and loud noises can be heard on the grounds after dark," warns a writer on spookyplaces.us. There are also reports of a large orb that chases people around, and sightings of apparitions wondering the area. (64)

Abandoned since 2003, its most striking feature may be the small red and white sign, nailed to a stake in the ground at the edge of the property, which reads: FOR SALE BY OWNER. (There are no takers.)

There are, however, those who take a more reasoned, academic view of the asylum's decay, as expressed by Gerald Grob, Ph.D., a former professor of medical history at Rutgers University, whose books on the topic include *The Mad among Us: A History of the Care of America's mentally Ill.* "Those buildings are a great window into understanding how much differently society dealt with the problem of mental illness back in the day." (65)

Well, 'back in the day' is a subject worth exploring.

Insanity

In fact, the meaning of the term insanity, itself, was much debated for decades, as evidenced by a paper presented at the American Medico Psychological Association at the Fifty-Eighth Annual Meeting held in 1902. The treatise was offered by E. Stanley Allot, M. D., formerly of Mclean Hospital in Boston. One of the oldest psychiatric hospitals in America, Mclean pre-dates the New York institutions by more than 50 years. (66)

Hudson River Hospital for the Insane

The main points of the paper were quite basic.

"The rapid spread in recent years of the desire to study the insane by modern scientific methods, as shown by the establishment of laboratories and the appointment of specially qualified assistants, leads us to ask, at what kind of problems should we work? In what
Order should we attack them, and by what methods for work according to the laws of logic? The methods of work will suggest and develop themselves when we have once clearly defined what the problem is. It is the purpose of this paper, therefore, to indicate the nature of the legitimate problems of psychiatry, and to show their natural order and their relations to each other and to the general medical sciences.
"Although in the biological order cause precedes effect, and it would therefore seem more logical to study etiology before symptomatology, we must remember that it is the effect (of insanity) which comes first to our notice, and that we cannot study causes except in the light of effects. Therefore it is that the first problem is not what causes insanity, but what is insanity? And if we can clearly define this, we are in a better position to attack the problems of causation. In fact, our present ignorance of the causes of insanity is largely due to our ignorance of what insanity really is. The effort, then, to define insanity has not merely an academic or medico-legal interest, but is essential to a thorough scientific study of the subject. Our efforts may not meet with success, but that does not excuse us from trying. Each sincere effort brings us a little nearer the truth, until finally someone will state it in a form that will receive general recognition." (67)

In point of fact, while insanity was neither understood nor well-defined during the first decades of the Hudson River Asylum's operation, it was also not a requirement for commitment. According to Roger Christianson, Director of the Hudson River Psychiatric Hospital Museum, only about 1/3 of the patients at the asylum was thought to be mentally ill. Most of the residents were there simply because they needed a place to live, and the ways they got there were many and varied. In the first instance, a person could simply walk up to the asylum or be dropped off by their family and that was sufficient for admission. Likewise, elderly parents were often taken there; husbands dropped off their shrewish wives, wives of drunk or abusive husbands could have them committed by signing a form, and unruly teenagers could be left there by their parents. People with money were often taken there by greedy family members who sought control of their estates. Anyone with a grudge against another could initiate commitment.

While one might expect the New York Times to be an excellent resource for researching the history of the Hudson River Asylum that is unfortunately not the case. Like the state of New York which has sealed all documents relating to this institution (with a few rare exceptions) newspaper archives of the region are almost completely devoid of any information on Hudson. But there were exceptions.

The New York Times

Published: February 12, 1889
Women Sent to Insane Asylum.
Rondout, N.Y. Feb. 11.This afternoon Police Captain T. Reilly of New York took his sister-in-law, Mrs. Catherine Reilly, to the Hudson River Insane Asylum at Poughkeepsie. For several days she has acted as though demented, muttering something to the effect that the "White Caps "were pursuing her. Mrs. O'Reilly has lived here for many years and is generally respected.

The New York Times

Published: March 16, 1895
POUGHKEEPSIE, NY., March 15.R.J. Ryan an insane patient, escaped from the Hudson River State Hospital at Rhinecliff stealing lights from the signal posts on the Hudson River Railroad. He was brought back to the asylum this morning

The New York Times

September 6, 1903
POUKEEPSIE, Sept 5.On Complaint of Superintendent Charles W. Pilgrim of the Hudson

River State Hospital, Frank A. Sanders, an attendant, was held today for the Grand Jury on the charge of misusing John Hayes, a patient, while Hayes lay helpless on a bed under what is called a protection sheet, which is used in cases of suicidal mania.

Sanders is said to have confessed that while intoxicated he amused himself by ticking the feet and ribs of Mr. Hayes. Sanders said that if he had been sober none of this would have happened and he is very sorry for what he has done.

Mr. I.G. Harris who is over the ward where Hayes is confined stated today that Sanders will be prosecuted to the full extent of the law, as an example to other attendants, and other asylums. (68)

Not well mentally

Frederic Mors, an Austrian immigrant, has the unique distinction of having been a patient in three of New York's insane asylums. His tale is a cautionary one.

Born Carl Menarik in 1889, Frederic Mors immigrated to the United States and settled in New York City. Assuming the name, Frederic Mors, he soon finds employment at the German Old Fellows Home in the Bronx, as an orderly. Almost immediately Mors begins acting in a strange manner, telling patients he is a doctor and demanding to be referred to as 'Herr Doktor' and that he was also a 'legendary hunter'.

Mors may have begun killing soon after his arrival at the home but nothing was suspected for six months. But soon, many 'suspicious' deaths of elderly patients began to occur. Mors was confronted and immediately confessed. Without hesitation, Mors admitted that he had 'perfected' a method of dispensing chloroform poisoning. He stated he had done so in order to put the 'old folks' out of their misery and to make room for others in the crowded home. Mors went on to say he had killed approximately seventeen patients in that manner.

Upon his confession, Mors was sent to Bellevue Hospital for a mental evaluation. The examination revealed him to be, "not well mentally" and he was committed to Hudson River Hospital for the Insane for a further examination. While at Hudson River he was found by jury to be criminally insane and was committed to Matteawan Hospital for the Criminally Insane.

After several years at Matteawan, Mors escaped. It was said that he "just walked away". Mors was never caught but authorities appeared to take his escape in stride stating he was not "considered dangerous". Mors, as far as we know, disappeared into obscurity, never to be heard from again. (69)

***

The Hudson River Asylum for the Chronic Insane was a self-contained community where people lived and worked in support of their own care. Treatment, such as it was, consisted of the occupational therapy of living life and participating in the support the essential needs of the community. Patients worked as farmers, bakers, butchers, seamstresses, milliners, furniture makers, and general laborers--all in support of the community. It was a place where people lived, worked, and played. There were recreation facilities—billiard rooms, athletic fields, walking paths—there were sports teams, picnics, clubs, even a marching band which was popular in the town of Poughkeepsie. This

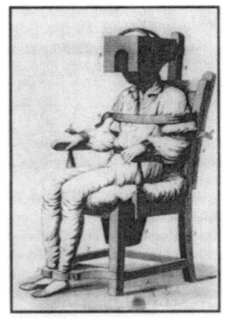

Holding Chair. A restraining device that led to many serious abuses, including torture and death.

was the heyday of "moral treatment" for the mentally ill, the disadvantaged, and the destitute. It lasted barely 30 years.

Unfortunately, the success of this institution, and others like it, led to ever increasing numbers of patients until "patient management" became the major preoccupation of staff and administration. This gave rise to the more widely known methods of handling the mentally ill in the first half of the 20th-century. Restraint, isolation, deprivation, pharmacological management, shock treatment, lobotomies, and the like, eventually became the dominant treatment modalities of their time. Ultimately, the "community" became too big, and the whole thing imploded and the model began to slip into history. (70)

Chapter 13
Buffalo Asylum for the Insane

The most distinctive features of the Buffalo State Asylum for the Insane are the two sprawling towers, thrusting towards the sky in medieval defiance. One look at this mansion-like compound, known today as the H.H. Richardson Complex, and you could easily think you have seen it as the backdrop to the opening credits of any number of low-budget horror films staring Christopher Lee or Vincent Price.

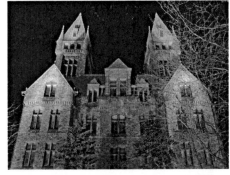

But the events that took place within these walls were not part of any movie script, and in fact, the design, while evocative of Bram Stocker's Transylvania, was actually meant to create an environment that was intended to provide the insane with a sense of security and well-being.

Buffalo State is a prime example of a Kirkbride Building – conceived by Pennsylvania's Dr. Thomas Story Kirkbride, (see

Buffalo State Asylum for the Insane was designed in 1870 in the "Kirkbride" Plan by architect Henry Hobson Richardson. Today many claim it is haunted.

Chapter One for Kirkbride's biography) which became the standard blueprint for the asylums built to house the mentally ill and criminally insane throughout the northeast in the nineteenth century. Kirkbride's ideas, espoused in his landmark, *On the Construction, Organization and General Arrangements of Hospitals for the Insane* were to provide a "moral alternative" for the insane, tucked away in a picturesque setting, far from the norms of society, where they could receive proper care. (71)

Kirkbride and his contemporaries saw these "Insane Asylums" as places that offered a chance at life for inmates, that they could not receive at home or anywhere else. Here, removed from society, in a place of relative protection, the insane were free to be as mad as they wanted or needed to be. In theory, they were also given the opportunity, for at least some of them, to work through their madness and return to sanity and mental stability.

However, like many ground-breaking concepts regarding the care and treatment of the mentally ill during the mid-to late 1800's, what started out with the best of intentions, soon fell into a downward spiral, due to overcrowding, lack of funding, abuse, and mismanagement -- but more on that later.

The Hospital's buildings were actually designed by Henry Hobson Richardson, as were many similar state asylums for the insane built at that time throughout the region. Interestingly enough, Richardson also designed many of the State Capital buildings in Albany –(the reader may draw his or her own conclusions about what that may say about the mental states of NY politicians then and now).

Construction on the asylum began in 1870, and the central administration buildings, those two iconic towers, and a number of flanking pavilions to house patients, were completed in 1880, and the facility opened. Final construction was not completed until 1895.

The Buffalo State Hospital was closed to the public and patients in 1974. Today, the hospital is off-limits to all except those responsible for what little routine maintenance the buildings still receive. Yet those who have dared enter the site have risked more than a breaking and entering charge. The Buffalo State Asylum is listed as one of New York's most haunted places, and has been the site of several paranormal investigations. (72)

Tales of Abuse and Cruelty

Certainly, as with many of the asylums of the times, there were reports of cruelty and abuse at Buffalo. A New York Times article dated March 3 of 1881, for example, spoke of a complaint brought to the State Commissioner in

Lunacy, by an attendant, about two fellow attendants who he witnessed to have "habitually maltreated patients in their care." Another Times article dated, February 7th the same year was more specific about the same two attendants, named Jones and McMichael. This article stated that McMichael had been witnessed to choke, almost drown, and severely beat patients to "keep them quiet." (73)

Understand, however, allegations of this kind aside, many of the practices that we now recognize as barbaric or cruel, were actually thought to be legitimate treatments, even cures for mental illness back in late 19th century. One such gruesome practice was eugenics, or the idea of intentionally sterilizing insane patients so that they would not be able to have offspring and pass on their "bad seed."

In addition to the typical bed restraints and straight jackets that were also considered "treatment" at the time, schizophrenics were routinely injected with insulin to starve their brains of so much sugar that only the most "primitive" functions remained inducing a kind of "chemical lobotomy." To be sure, many physical lobotomies and other forms of barbaric experimental brain surgery were likely also performed on patients at the asylum.

A Haunted Past

Many of those that study the paranormal believe that the alleged haunting of places such as Buffalo State occurs because the tortured and unsettled state these folks endured in life translates into a tortured and unsettled afterlife. Are those who were sent to Buffalo State because they were deemed unworthy to live amongst us in life – now still bound to the place, lying there still tied in restraints and straight jackets, equally unworthy of entering the hereafter?

There have been many reports of unusual sights and sounds in and around the grounds of the hospital by nearby Buffalo State College students, many of whom have ventured illegally onto the property.

According to several paranormal investigators, students have reported hearing screams and slamming doors coming from the grounds. There have also been reports of "demonic figures" moving by the windows of former patient rooms.

Whether such reports are true or just typical of those associated with "spooky places," a visit to the Hospital is creepy by any stretch of the imagination. Students who have snuck in have described an instantaneous and almost overwhelming feeling of dread.

There are several videos on the internet, made by "professional" and amateur paranormal investigators alike, who have entered the property that purport to capture paranormal activity going on at the asylum. The best known of these is the "Haunted Film" made by an anonymous paranormal investigator known only as Dave. Dave gave the film to the Friends of Endangered History, and it can be viewed on their website, hauntedfilm.com, where you may draw your own conclusions. (74)

Halloween at Murder Creek

The most infamous "ghost story" surrounding The Buffalo State Asylum involved the case of Sadie (Sarah) McMullen and is known as "Halloween at Murder Creek." As the story goes, on Halloween 1890, Sadie McMullen in a fit of insane rage threw two children, Delia Brown, Age 6 and Nellie May Connors age 8, off of the railroad bridge over Murder Creek in Akron, N.Y. Sadie then attempted to take her own life by also jumping from the bridge.

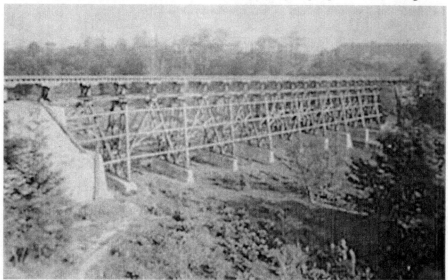

"Halloween at Murder Creek" involved the strange case of Sadie McMullen who threw two small girls off a railroad trestle, killing one of them. She went to trial and was found 'not guilty by reason of insanity'. She spent eighteen months at the Buffalo Asylum.

Nellie died, but Delia survived. According to testimony she said to the rescuer who found her: "Sarah thought she was really smart to throw us off of the bridge didn't she?"

What exactly the little girl meant by those words remains a mystery. Had Sadie been convicted of murder, she would have been the first woman to be put to death in NY using the recently introduced electric chair.

After trial, Sadie was committed to Buffalo State for two-years. After she was released, she vanished without a trace and was never seen or heard from again... or was she? (75)

According to area legend, the ghost of Sadie returns every Halloween to join the others that stalk the now abandoned corridors of The Buffalo State Asylum.

***

Whether Buffalo State and places like it are haunted by ghosts, or just the echoes of the darkness of turn-of-the century medical thinking, depends on your perspective. But in any case it should stand as a tribute to the souls who suffered and died there, and to those who did try to help them.

Chapter 14

Middletown State Homeopathic Hospital

Middletown State Homeopathic Hospital located in Middletown New York opened on April 20, 1874 with 69 patients. It was the first pure homeopathic hospital established for mental disorders in the United States. The push for state homeopathic institutions for the treatment of mental disorders began just eight years earlier in 1875, John Stanton-Gould delivered a speech to the State Homeopathic Medical Society

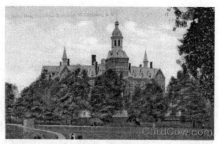

Middletown State Homeopathic Hospital located in Middletown, New York, was the first purely homeopathic hospital for mental disorders in the United States.

entitled 'The Relation of Insanity to Bodily Disease'. In this speech, Gould asserted that "It has been my purpose in this address, gentlemen, to bring before you in a clear and specific form the proofs that insanity is always a symptom of bodily disease which it is your duty and ought to be your pleasure to cure." At the next meeting of the State Homeopathic Medical Society, they passed a resolution to push the New York State Legislature to construct an institution for the treatment of mental disorders along homeopathic lines. The state legislature approved a bill for the establishment of a state hospital in Middletown to use homeopathic therapy methods.

Henry Reed Stiles became the second superintendent of the hospital in 1875 and introduced strict dietary regimens. From 1877 until 1902, Dr. Seldon H. Talcott was the superintendent and developed a series of occupational therapy for all patients at Middletown. His treatment included art exhibitions, an institutional newsletter written by the patients (The Conglomerate), and athletics including baseball. But the origins of homeopathy as a means to treat the mentally ill had begun many years earlier with the work of Samuel Hahnemann. (76)

Origins of Homeopathy

Samuel Hahnemann was a German physician, linguist, and scholar living in the early 1800's who was frustrated with the medicine of his time. He noticed that medicine often had the effect of making patients sicker, whether immediately or at a later time. While studying the writings of a British scientist, he rediscovered the principle "like cures like." Intrigued by what he read, Hahnemann gave himself heavy doses of quinine (used to treat malaria), finding to his amazement that he came down with malarial symptoms.

He experimented with nearly 100 substances throughout his life, "proving" their capacity to cure the same symptoms that they produced in healthy human subjects. He found that when the energy of these particular substances had been "captured," they were able to cure the same symptoms (not necessarily the same illness) that were produced by ingesting the crude form. By a process of dilution of the "mother tincture" - the original extract - followed by potentiating (energizing through shaking called succession), homeopathic remedies were created. Many American MDs added to our understanding of remedy "states" (non-optimum mental or physical states) such as Kent, Herring, Clarke, and George Vithoulkas produced a scientific explanation of homeopathy.

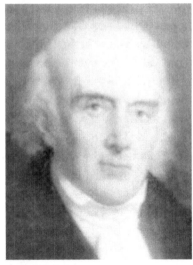

Samuel Hahnemann (1755-1843) was a German physician, best known for creating a system of alternative medicine called homeopathy that was used for the treatment of mental illnesses.

Middletown State Homeopathic Hospital

The Science of Healing

Through many years of study and experimentation, Hahnemann discovered that true healing is possible only by allowing the body's innate wisdom to direct the course of recovery. He found this was best achieved by medicine which produced a cure from the inside out. This concept contrasted directly with the allopathic view (standard medicine) which aimed to suppress or control symptoms and declare it a cure. It was Hahnemann's observation that allopathic medicines drove the physiological condition towards a deeper pathology because the body's own intelligence had been "turned off." We might name that intelligence vital force; in its physical form it is immunity.

For instance, children given creams for rashes later developed allergies, which when suppressed became asthma. Adults treated for sexually transmitted diseases became mentally and emotionally disturbed. And so on and so forth; the more suppressive treatment, the more serious the health condition of the individual became.

Can homeopathy cure mental illness?

It was felt that although this question probably couldn't be answered, it was believed that with a well-chosen remedy, tendencies could be diminished. Homeopathy was believed by its adherents, to have at least the potential to change the very cellular mechanisms of the nervous system. This could have a particularly significant impact on children and on adults who planned to have children in terms of preventing the genetic expression of undesirable behaviors and pathology. (77)

Baseball Therapy

Dr. Talcott's progressive, and some might say, unorthodox ideas about how to treat the mentally ill, was radically different than what was then being practiced, namely the warehousing of the insane in asylums and poorhouses. Talcott believed a healthy mind should reside in a healthy body (homeopathy). As he put it, "the physical means for recuperating the worn and wasted systems of the insane may be stated in three words—heat, milk, and rest, and the greatest of these is rest." Talcott and his staff at Middletown also believed in stimulating patients' minds through activities. The hospital had educational classes, theater, and its own patient-run newspaper. The doctors also encouraged their wards to exercise, in the fresh air if possible, and soon settled upon the before mentioned playing of baseball as a way to give male inmates a workout and provide a sort of therapy to other patients who could become attentive fans and focus on the game instead of their troubles.

Baseball, the sole nationally popular team sport in America at the time, was not a new tool for mental health practitioners. Its usefulness in treatment had been known of for years, but the Middletown staff went a step farther. In 1888, they founded a team partially composed of patients, hospital employees, and some of the best local amateurs and semiprofessionals, to be an informal part of the treatment regimen. That didn't last long because the team soon developed into a semipro powerhouse in the lower-Hudson River Valley area north of New York City, and thousands came to see its marquee games.

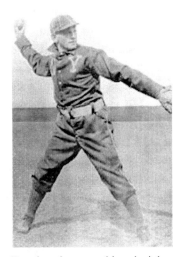

Based on homeopathic principles, Middletown State Hospital founded a baseball team comprised of patients, staff and amateur baseball players. The team was called, "The Asylums". Jack Chesboro pictured here, started his career playing for Middletown Hospital.

The team began play in 1889 as the "Asylums" and played other teams in the region. By 1890, the team was playing regional teams from New York City and elsewhere, winning 21 games out of 25, including the Cuban Giants, one of the top baseball teams at the time. In 1891, they narrowly lost a game with the New York Giants who had finished 3rd in the National League that year, 4-3. In 1892, the team went undefeated except for two narrow losses to the New York Giants, again defeating the Cuban Giants, and many other teams from New York and New Jersey. Over the next few years, a number of excellent semi-pro players played for the Asylums were recruited directly from the Asylums to professional baseball.(78) One of those ball players, who went on to a hall of fame career, was John 'Jack' Chesbro. (79) John 'Happy Jack' Chesbro, (real name Chesebrough, whose name was shortened by a sports writer so his name would fit into the box score) would win 41 games

Middletown State Homeopathic Hospital

in the 1904 season which remains an MLB record to this day and is viewed as unbreakable. He was given the nick name, 'Happy Jack' by a Middletown patient due to his pleasant demeanor. (80)

***

The number of buildings at Middletown would eventually reach over 100 and the number of patients grew to 2,250 by the early 1900s and 3,686 patients by the 1960s. Gradually though, the emphasis of the hospitals services began to shift in the latter half of the 1970's and 80's primarily to outpatient therapy and inpatient numbers decreased. The institution permanently closed in 2006. (81)

Chapter 15

Matteawan State Hospital for the Criminally Insane

Matteawan State Hospital for the Criminally Insane, as well as those asylums that came before its inception in 1892, evolved painfully over the course of this nation's history, filling a burgeoning need to care for the criminally mentally ill. From the almshouses of the 17th and 18th century to the squalid quarters that confined so many, the treatment of the mentally ill criminal evolved from a philosophy of containing "moral depravity".(82)

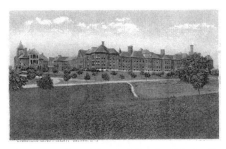

Matteawan State Hospital for the Criminally Insane would hold convicted and un-convicted criminals (?) Including both men and women.

Reform

By the 1820s early reforms began with the likes of Thomas Eddy, treasurer of New York Hospital, and later in the 1840s with Dorothea Dix, who stressed humane care of those afflicted with mental illness, even those deemed to be criminals. These early pioneers held up a mirror to the world of overcrowded, understaffed asylums rife with frequent and terrible epidemics, corrupt administrations, and endless human suffering. (83)

Matteawan State Hospital for the Criminally Insane

Images of neglected inmates lost in their own despair proved to be too much for even literary giant, Charles Dickens, who upon a visit to a New York City asylum was appalled and haunted for the rest of his life by the abject conditions he observed.(84)

One of the earliest institutions for the criminally insane in New York was located in Auburn, the county seat of Cayuga County. Known as The New York State Lunatic Asylum for Insane Convicts, this was the first structure designed specifically to house convicted criminals deemed to be insane. Previously, they were detained in prisons, hospitals, and in some cases almshouses.

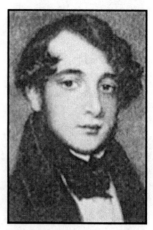

Charles Dickens (1812-1890) upon visiting an insane asylum, was alleged to have commented "What I saw was naked ugliness and horror".

Auburn Prison

In addition being an asylum for the criminally insane, Auburn was also the site of the oldest existing state correctional facility. The cornerstone for this 10-acre prison was laid in 1816 and in 1817 it housed 53 prisoners. In future years it would accommodate as many as 700 inmates. To this day, the prison is open although its name was changed in 1970 to The Auburn Correctional Facility.

Auburn, with its constant source of waterpower, was an ideal location for a prison and convict labor. It was used for shoemaking, cabinetry, tool making, and in the nearby woolen mills. This facility was the first in the nation to use separate cells for inmates and it greatly influenced the subsequent construction of many similar prisons in other states. (85)

The Electric Chair

Auburn prison made notorious history on August 6, 1890 when the nation's very first execution by electric chair took place. William Kemler was found guilty of murdering his common law wife, Matilda "Tillie" Ziegler, with a hatchet and sentenced to death by electrocution.

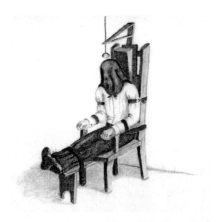

William Kemmler (1860-1890) from Buffalo, New York, was a convicted murderer and the first person to be executed using the electric chair. He did not die quickly.

His lawyers tried to appeal the court's decision on the grounds that it was cruel and unusual punishment. Powerful patrons such as business magnate, George Westinghouse (the appliance guy), supported the cry for appeal, but it failed partially because Thomas Edison supported the state's decision.

Kemler did not die the first time around and a second volt of electricity was required. According to the New York Herald, his death was hideous to behold and "strong men fainted and fell like logs on the floor" as they viewed his writhing and suffering, smelled his flesh burning and watched in horror as smoke curled up from his head.(86)

In the spring of 1892, the Auburn Asylum for Insane Convicts moved to the former site of the 246-acre Dates Farm, which was situated in the village of Matteawan in Fishkill, New York, between the Hudson River and the rolling Fishkill Mountains. It was then renamed Matteawan State Hospital. (87)

Architect, Isaac Perry, known as the first state architect in New York, was hired to design the main hospital building with "an abundance of light and ventilation" that would be able to accommodate up to 550 patients. He was chosen because of his stellar reputation; Governor Grover Cleveland had personally selected Perry to put the finishing touches on the New York State Capitol building.

Matteawan was originally intended to house patients that were too dangerous for civilian institutions such as Utica Asylum, Hudson River State Hospital, and too ill for other prisons such as Sing Sing. Security was tighter than elsewhere, but except for that Matteawan functioned exactly like other hospitals housing the insane.

Patients at Matteawan were awarded some amenities. They were able to exercise outdoors in the courtyards twice a day and to participate in sporting activities such as: softball, tennis, bowling, shuffleboard, volleyball, chess, checkers, card games, gymnastics, ping pong and a version of horse-shoes called quoits. Later in the 1900's, the wards were equipped with radios and phonographs and on special occasions, such as Christmas, vaudeville shows were staged for the patients.

Due to the fact that the inmate population of Matteawan constantly increased, it was just a matter of time before the institution's 550 beds became insufficient to house them. In 1899, another prison mental health hospital was built on the grounds of Clinton County in the village of Dannemora, New York. (88)

Eventually Matteawan State Hospital transferred all of its male inmates who had at least six months left to serve on their sentences to Dannemora State Hospital as well as all males serving sentences for felonies and who were declared insane. Female inmates who fell into both of these categories were retained at Matteawan.

Arguably two of the most notorious patient/prisoners ever confined in Matteawan were Lizzie Halliday "The worst woman on earth", and Harry Thaw and "the trial of the century."

Harry Thaw and the "Trial of the Century"

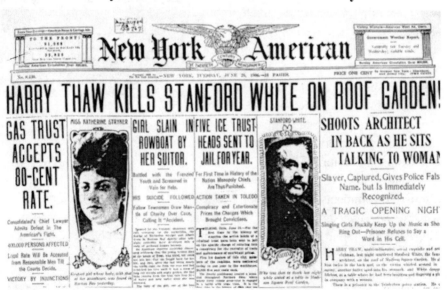

"It had wealth, degeneracy, young chorus girls, the Underworld, the Great White Way, and madness-Irvine Cobb, reporter for New York American.

One of the most notorious inmates of the Matteawan Hospital for the Criminally Insane was millionaire Harry Thaw, who was incarcerated in the mental hospital in 1908 after killing architect Stanford White. Thaw's story is one of jealousy, scandal, intrigue and possibly feigned insanity.

History of Tension Between Henry Thaw and Stanford White

Thaw was the son of a wealthy coal and railroad baron. Troubled and known for various kinds of bad behavior from the time he was a child, Thaw grew up to lead a life of hedonism, known by many as a "playboy." Thaw dabbled heavily in various vices, including hardcore drugs, serious gambling, cockfighting, alcohol abuse, and chasing after women, particularly showgirls. His profligate lifestyle was funded by his wealthy parents.

Thaw met and quickly formed a rivalry with architect Stanford White through their mutual interest in showgirls and the partying lifestyle. Thaw and White ran in some of the same circles, but White was generally considered much more respectable and achieved a high level of social stature that remained out of reach for Thaw. When Thaw's money was not enough to keep him from being rejected by various high-class social clubs in New York City, all of which refused his membership, Thaw blamed Stanford White rather than his own bad behavior.

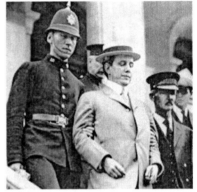

Harry Kendall Thaw (1871-1947) Plagued by mental illness since childhood, was convicted of murder in the "trial of the century." He spent nine years in the Matteawan Asylum for the Criminally Insane.

Thaw also blamed White, and dismissive comments he'd allegedly made about Thaw, for his lack of success with wooing various showgirls. This jealous rivalry all came to a head when Thaw met and fell in love with White's sometime lover, Evelyn Nesbit.

Troubled Relationship with "The Girl in the Red Velvet Swing"

Evelyn Nesbit was a beautiful young showgirl known as "the girl in the red velvet swing." This nickname was based on rumors that Stanford White had a red velvet swing hanging from the ceiling in his home, in which he would seat Evelyn (and his other lovers) in order to lasciviously look up her skirts as she swung. Evelyn and White had an on-again-off-again relationship. Thaw became obsessed with Evelyn, partially thanks to her great beauty and partially thanks to his intense rivalry with White. White warned Evelyn to stay away from Thaw, but Thaw persisted and eventually wore down her defenses.

Thaw eventually convinced Evelyn to marry him, after taking Evelyn and her mother on an extravagant, months-long tour of Europe. After they were married, however, Thaw's obsession with Stanford White only seemed to increase. His

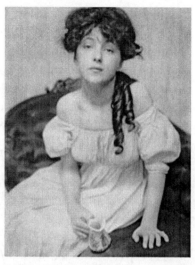

Evelyn Nesbit (1884-1967) popular chorus girl immortalized as, "The Girl in the Velvet Swing"

romantic, passionate wooing of Evelyn ended once they were married, and he instead became increasingly abusive. He would often beat and whip her, all the while forcing her to confess to various sexual acts she's engaged in with Stanford White. As time went on he became more and more irrationally angry with his former rival, to the point of complete obsession.

Thaw's Behavior Leading up to the Murder

On June 25, 1906, Harry Thaw, his wife Evelyn, and two friends attended a play being shown on the rooftop of Madison Square Gardens. His behavior in the hours before attending the play was bizarre, even for Thaw. He'd learned earlier that day that Stanford White was planning to attend the same play. Leaving Evelyn at their hotel, Thaw disappeared for a few hours without explanation. He returned in time to leave for the play, strangely insisting on wearing a long black overcoat, despite the warm summer weather. Evelyn noted that he was agitated and talking strangely, but by now she was accustomed to his odd behavior. Once at Madison Square Garden he emphatically refused to allow the coat check girl to take his black overcoat, insisting on wearing it to the play.

The Murder and Subsequent Trials

During the play, Thaw was seen approaching Stanford White's table and then backing away and returning to his own table several times. Finally, during the closing musical number of the play, Thaw enacted his plan. He walked up to White, pulled out the gun he'd concealed under his long black coat, and shot White three times in the face, point-blank. White was killed instantly. Some members of the audience initially thought the shooting wasn't real, but was rather a prank having to do with the play.

Thaw ended up having two separate murder trials. At the first trial, the jury was deadlocked and could not reach a verdict. At the second trial, Thaw pleaded non-guilty by reason of insanity. The murder and the two trials captured the imagination of the public at large, with people all over the United States obsessed with the sensationalistic headlines. The dramatic second trial came to be called the "Trial of the Century" and was reported in lurid detail in newspapers.

In order to demonstrate his insanity, Thaw insisted that Evelyn serve as a witness and thoroughly coached her on what to say. At Thaw's insistence, Evelyn claimed on the witness stand that Stanford White had been extremely abusive of her and that she feared for her life at his hands. Evelyn also claimed that Thaw only killed White in a moment of temporary insanity, in a misguided attempt to protect her. There is reason to believe that Evelyn only testified because she was promised by Thaw's mother that if she did so she would receive one million dollars and a divorce.

In any case, the jury was enchanted by Evelyn's beauty and her dramatic story. Thaw's insanity plea was accepted and he was incarcerated in the Matteawan Hospital for the Criminally Insane. Evelyn did receive her divorce, but not the million dollars. During Thaw's incarceration she gave birth to a son, whom she claimed was conceived during an illicit conjugal visit, but Thaw refused to admit he was the father. Evelyn ended up raising her son in relative poverty, with no access to the Thaw family wealth.

Thaw's Stay at Matteawan and his Escape to Quebec

By all accounts, thanks to his family's fortune and his own notoriety, Thaw's time at the Matteawan Hospital for the Criminally Insane was much more pleasant and unrestricted than it would have been if he were just a regular patient. Thaw was allowed a great deal of freedom in the hospital, and was well-treated. Despite the good treatment he received, however, Thaw began pushing for his own release almost immediately after becoming an inmate of the hospital. He attempted several times to be declared sane and allowed to leave, on the grounds that he was only accused of "temporary insanity."

Unfortunately for Thaw, his past caught up to him with many witnesses coming forward to tell the jury at his sanity trial tales of Thaw's frequently bizarre behavior. Unable to get the legal release from Matteawan he sought, Thaw took matters into his own hands and escaped the hospital in 1913. This escape was singularly un-dramatic, with Thaw reputedly just walking out of the hospital and getting into a hired car that took him across the border to Quebec. The ease of his escape can likely be explained by bribes for the hospital guards. In any case, Thaw made it to Quebec but was soon found and extradited back to the United States and sent back to the asylum. By this time he was considered something of a national folk hero. His 1915 sanity trial was much more successful than earlier attempts. At this time Thaw was officially declared sane by a jury and allowed to be released.

Post-script:

Thaw didn't suddenly become a mild-mannered, law-abiding citizen upon his release from the Matteawan Hospital for the Criminally Insane. In 1916, less than a year after his release, he was arrested for sexually assaulting and beating a young man. Thaw once again pleaded temporary insanity, and was once again locked up in a mental institution, this time the famous Kirkbride Asylum in Philadelphia. He was declared sane and released for good in 1924.

The Worst Woman on Earth

Lizzie Halliday is one of the most remarkable psychopathic killers in American criminal history. Born with the desire to kill, she exacted a heavy toll of lives before she was finally sent to Matteawan Hospital for the Criminally Insane and even there murdered an attendant and attempted to murder another by stabbing her more than 200 times in the face with a pair of scissors. Halliday, was simply known as, "the worst woman on earth".

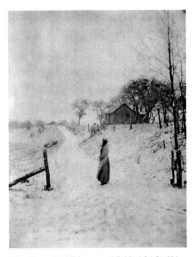

Lizzie Halliday (1860-1918). Was confined for twenty-five years at Matteawan State Hospital. Was considered, "among the worst type of the criminal insane".

She was Elizabeth Mcnally, born in Ireland in 1861, and came to America in 1887, where she married Charles Hopkins. Hopkins died suddenly under suspicious circumstances.

Lizzie then married Artemas Brewster. He died within a year. She then married Hiram Parkinson, from who she separated. George Smith became her next husband. After trying to poison him she fled to Bellows Falls, Vt. For two weeks, she became the wife of Charles Pleystein until he fled, some say, fearing for his life.

Lizzie was later convicted of burning down a small store in Philadelphia for the insurance money and served two years in the penitentiary. Later in Newburgh, New York she married Paul Halliday, a septuagenarian with an imbecile son. Her first step was to set fire to the Halliday home, burning to death her newly acquired step-son.

In 1893 Mr. Halliday disappeared. A search of the cellar revealed the bodies of Margaret McQuinlan and her daughter, Sarah. A day or two later her husband's body was found buried under the house. She was also suspected of having murdered a peddler named Hutch some time earlier. The total number of her victims remains unknown.

Her sentence of death was eventually commuted after a commission of doctors had pronounced her insane. She spent the rest of her life confined to a cell and manacled to her wall. (90)

Chapter 16
Bloomingdale Insane Asylum

Unlike the public, state-funded mental hospitals that sprung up across the country in the mid-19th century, the Bloomingdale Insane Asylum was privately funded and operated. The asylum was built on the same land in what is currently upper Manhattan's Morningside Heights neighborhood that now houses Columbia University. At the time the institution was built, the area was a rural, pastoral countryside. The land purchased for the asylum stretched from 110th to 120th Streets and from Riverside Drive to Morningside Drive. Funding for the hospital came from charitable contributions to a fund called the Society of the New York Hospital.

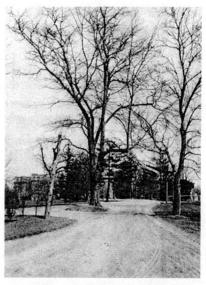

Bloomingdale Private hospital for the care of the mentally ill located in the Morningside Heights area of NYC now occupied by Columbia University

Thomas Eddy, a prominent Quaker banker and a vocal advocate for better treatment of the mentally ill, led the Society's search for land for the new asylum. (91)

Beginning in 1816 the society purchased 26 acres of land in Manhattan for the hospital project. By 1821 the large, elegant Federal-style hospital building had been constructed on the land and was ready for operations to commence. The Bloomingdale Insane Asylum was created a couple of decades before the publicly-funded mental hospitals began opening across New York State and the rest of the country. Once this phenomenon took root, however, the asylum in Bloomingdale became a hospital almost exclusively for those patients with financially well-off families, since the poorer mentally ill could stay at the state-funded hospitals for free.

The Bloomingdale asylum, like many of its public counterparts, was surrounded by elegant, carefully laid out grounds and walkways. The designers of the grounds and the asylum itself placed a deliberate emphasis on wide open spaces where patients could feel at ease, rested, and unconfined. Patients could stroll around the grounds, taking in the peaceful scenery and gardens. There were also extensive orchards, vegetable gardens, and even a full working farm on which patients could perform moderate physical work, thought to be therapeutic.

The Bloomingdale asylum was intended to conform to the tenants of moral treatment, which was the more humane method of treating the mentally ill and which was beginning to gain ground in Europe and throughout the United States at the time. Moral treatment involved treating the patients in a kind and compassionate manner, without the use of shackles, chains, or other restraints, and allowed for plenty of therapeutic recreational and occupational activity, such as farm work, landscaping, painting, dancing and writing. Thus, the patients at the Bloomingdale asylum were initially treated quite well, and provided with ample healthy, fresh food, moderate exercise, and plenty of time for relaxation and rest, as well as sunshine. (92)

Julius Chambers Controversy

The Bloomingdale Insane Asylum's initial altruistic intentions and private funding did not protect it from accusations of abuse and neglect that were similar to those directed at many of the public mental institutions. While, like most of the 19th century asylums, the Bloomindale asylum began with the most benevolent of intentions, by the 1870's, overcrowding and rumors of rampant abuse became rising concerns. In 1872, an investigative reporter from the New

Bloomingdale Insane Asylum

York Tribune named Julius Chambers, assisted by many collaborators, decided to have himself committed to the asylum in order to perform an underground investigation of the facility. Chambers was assisted by his editors and friends in his successful attempt to get committed, and ended up spending a full ten days in the asylum before petitioning, with the help of his friends, to be released.

Once inside the institution, Chambers learned that the allegations of abuse, which had been widely whispered about in the community, barely touched upon the severity of the actual abuse. According to Chambers' first-hand account, patients at the Bloomingdale asylum were routinely choked, punched, and kicked, and some were even tormented so thoroughly by the staff that they were driven to suicide.

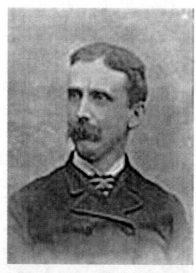

Julius Chambers (1850-1920) American author, editor, journalist and activist against psychiatric abuse. Had himself committed to Bloomingdale Asylum in order to write expose alleging maltreatment.

Chambers was completely horrified by much that he witnessed during his ten days inside the asylum, including what he believed to be the forced captivity of several patients whom he believed to be mentally stable and healthy, and not in need of institutionalization at all.

After Chambers petitioned the court to be released, having gathered all the information he needed, he wrote a series of expose style articles about the asylum that were published by the New York Tribune. These articles, detailing the abuses he witnessed during his stay at the asylum, shocked the public and led to court proceedings against the hospital. The articles ultimately led to 12 inmates of the asylum being released on the grounds that they were not insane and had been held in the asylum against their wills. The articles also led to major restructuring of the asylum, with those staff and administrators thought to be responsible for the abuses being fired. Ultimately Chambers' investigation of The Bloomingdale Insane Asylum helped lead to changes in the lunacy laws, making it more difficult for perfectly sane people to be held in mental institutions. (93)

Chambers' stories and articles were eventually published as a book called *A Mad World and Its Inhabitants*. After his book was published Chambers remained a life-long activist for the reform of the poor treatment of the mentally ill. He was often asked to speak about the rights of the mentally ill as well as what constituted humane and appropriate treatment and housing for them. He also continued to work as a journalist, as well as an editor and a travel writer. (94)

Artist Charles Deas

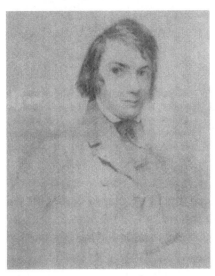

Charles Deas (1818-1867) artist best known for his oil paintings of Native Americans. In 1848 he was declared legally insane and institutionalized at Bloomingdale Asylum for the rest of his life.

American oil painter Charles Deas was institutionalized at Bloomingdale Insane Asylum from 1848 until his death in 1867. Deas was mainly known for his oil paintings of Native Americans, fur trappers, and other scenes from frontier life. After being born and raised in Philadelphia, and later living in New York, Deas decided to explore the American west in an attempt to emulate his painting mentor George Catlin. His extensive travels through the western territories and frontier provided much of the subject matter for his paintings. Deas spent months at a time living among Native American tribes near Saint Louis, Missouri, becoming intimately acquainted with their lifestyle and studying them closely, which allowed his painting to be highly realistic and personal. Common themes in Deas' paintings included struggle, tension, danger, and both implied and actual violence. One of his better known paintings depicted a fur trapper and a Native American locked together in combat, while plummeting to their deaths by falling from a cliff. (95)

The emotional and psychological intensity present in Deas' work was probably indicative of psychological difficulties and mental health issues, in addition to artistic talent. In 1848 he returned to New York City from his travels out west with the stated intention of opening an art gallery specializing in Native American art. Before he was able to do so, however, he was declared legally insane (under seemingly unknown circumstances) and committed to the Bloomingdale asylum. During the more than twenty years Deas was committed to the Bloomingdale asylum, he continued to create art. His oil paintings during this time were thought to be especially dark, intense, and in some cases, even disturbing, when compared to his earlier work. Deas was one of those rare artists

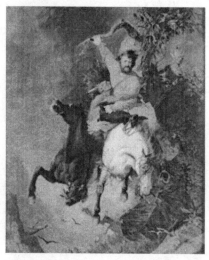

"The Death Struggle" by Charles Deas. His indisputable masterpiece.

who was much more famous when he was alive than after his death, having been relatively well-known during his life before being institutionalized and then becoming largely unknown after his death. However, in recent years Deas' work has unexpectedly received renewed attention. A recent exhibit at the Denver Museum of Art, called "Charles Deas and 1840's America," focused on exposing Deas' work to a new generation of art lovers who have most likely never heard of him. (96)

Legacy of the Bloomingdale Insane Asylum

By the 1880's, the trustees from the Society of the New York Hospital began selling off some of the land and buildings belonging to the asylum. At this point in New York City's history, the city was beginning to expand north into current-day Manhattan, so it made financial sense to do so. This move was also a good idea because by this time the patient population at the Bloomingdale asylum had grown so much that a larger site was thought to be needed. In 1892 the trustees of Columbia College, which later became Columbia University, bought the majority of the asylum's lands and buildings in order to build a new campus on the premises. The Bloomingdale asylum moved to its new, larger location in White Plains. This legacy of assisting those with mental health issues in the area continues in the behavioral health department of the modern-day New York Hospital.

Conclusion

S he is known simply as Miss X. Presumably, she had a name at one time; she had a family, a childhood, a life. Then, at the age of thirteen, she was dropped off at an asylum by persons unknown where she would spend the rest of her life. The year was 1885. Incredibly, she would remain a patient for the next 73 years of her life. She of course could not know that her life would span profound changes in the care of the mentally ill. This began with the movement towards treatment in large state-run institutions during the nineteenth-century and culminated with the de-institutionalization movement and the creation of the community mental health system that began at around the time of her death in 1958.

Notes, written in longhand and attached to her yellowed admissions papers, report, *"Shows loss of memory . . . Derangement now manifested began on religious subjects . . . She literally believes the Sunday-school lessons". Cause of insanity: 'Sincerity and love of truth, and finding that nearly everything was a lie.'" Another note in her surprisingly thin file reads, ". . . Has seemed peculiar all her life, always solitary, very quiet . . . never in play with other children . . . did not learn very quick . . . worried over studies . . . has not learned as much as others . . . very particular and slow . . . worries over food . . . thinks she is covered with bugs . . . insisted there was a river to cross . . . thinks mother is against her."* (97)

Nowadays Miss X's illness might be called schizophrenia and an effort would be made to treat her. Her "acute mania" went untreated though and got worse over the years. From her records: *"Very disorderly and untidy "... nervous and tears her clothing ... she has to be fed."*. Later: *"Unchanged"*. *"Received a rubber doll for Christmas and seemed quite pleased with it." "Never rational enough to do any chores, she spent most of her time rocking in a chair."*

"This is a striking example of how expensive it can be in terms of both human life and money not to provide treatment for mental patients," said John M. Anderson, a mental health advocate, on the occasion of her 70th anniversary at the institution. "If there had been good psychiatric treatment for this patient when she was first admitted, the chances are she could have spent her life as a normal person." Seventy years after her admission at the age of 83 Miss X was a shrunken little woman, a pitiful wretch, a chronic bystander to a life gone by. There was no celebration of the occasion of her anniversary. Miss X just sat, rocking in her chair. (98)

Most of the institutions, at the time of her admission, did not initially engage in treatment for the mentally ill. These were places that people went to for a variety of reasons, and once they entered, they rarely if ever came out. In New York, in the late 19th century, the "insane" included people prone to seizures, homosexuals, children with now what we call Down's syndrome and other mental handicaps, those accused of devil worship or witchcraft, of course, the 'mad', and, most often, the pauper class. It was believed that the mission of these institutions was the "removal of people from the worriment, the overwork, the unsanitary conditions and the unsuitable food of their homes, occupying body and mind in new employment, cheering the drooping and melancholy and soothing the excited and irritable." Patients who were able did useful work at the asylums, constructing new buildings, working on the farms or sewing. At that time, patients were admitted to the asylums only by court order. The more enlightened hospital directors held; "The insane are sick, not criminal," (99)

The Progressive Movement

During the latter half of the nineteenth century, New York asylums were at the leading edge of treatment of the mentally ill. At other times, the term "snake-pit" was used to describe them. There were horror stories about patients being abused, neglected, and even raped. One newspaper reporter told of seeing a

Conclusion

patient who had been confined in leather straps so long, their skin was growing around them. A common sight during those dark ages were patients (like Miss X) sitting in rocking chairs in hallways all day long, with no opportunity for activity. Some claimed having the patients work in the large garden areas during the day was therapeutic for them; others said they were used as slave labor to keep the hospital's food costs down. (100)

***

To a great extent, New York institutions mirrored other mental institutions of the time. They started out small, engaging in "moral treatment", and as they grew in population from the low hundreds into the thousands, treatment became harsher as budgets grew tighter. In the early part of the 20th century, some mental hospitals operated at the extreme end of the cruelty spectrum. Physical restraint was routinely employed. At times a significant many were confined to straitjackets. Particularly unruly patients were often chained to the walls and floors for days, months, even years at a time. Drug induced comas and electro-shock treatment became a frequent occurrence. Lobotomies were commonplace, and violence was rampant.

In 1913, the practice of forced castrations began. The Kansas Legislature passed a bill that allowed for criminals, idiots, epileptics, imbeciles and the insane to be subjected to what was politely called Eugenics. There was, however, nothing polite about the practice and as many as 1500 patients were rather brutally mutilated. Though castration diminished somewhat over the years, the procedure was not entirely abandoned until 1961. (101)

Congressional Investigations

In 1948, a scandal broke in the press over the deplorable conditions at many state institutions. Legal commitment papers couldn't be found for some of the patients, and some patients could not even be accurately identified. Many patients still were being admitted as a result of the legal process but weren't having their actual mental conditions evaluated by hospital officials. Record keeping in many states had all but ceased to exist.

In response to the charges, a Congressional panel was established to study the situation. After the committee released its report in October 1948,

Congress doubled Federal appropriations for state mental hospitals. The practice of placing patients in rocking chairs in hallways during the daytime was discontinued. Incidents of patient mistreatment were investigated and corrected. Psychiatrists from the Menninger Foundation volunteered some of their own time to examine patients nationally. (102)

In 1949, the first psychiatric social workers were hired. They began the first discharge plans for patients who were deemed ready for release. Social workers often had to acquaint patients with modern household appliances that didn't exist when they were admitted.

Patients began to receive outpatient treatment beginning in1951. In 1955 a major breakthrough was felt to have been achieved when psychotropic drugs were developed bringing hope to thousands and assisting in the diagnosis and treatment of some symptoms of mental disorders. In 1963, the President John F. Kennedy Community Mental Health Center Act led to the opening of community mental health centers (Arden Hill where I had worked was one of the first in New York). At that time Medicare and Medicaid were introduced as the Federal Government began to assume more responsibility for the cost of mental health care. In 1974, the Supplemental Security Income program (SSI) was implemented and state governments began to assume a greater role in the care of the elderly. During this period, professional staff was increased, including physicians and dentists to treat physical ailments. (103)

Community Mental Health System

Eventually, in the 1980s, managed care systems began to oversee the use of hospital care for psychiatric patients. Financial incentives presented by both public concerns and private insurance companies joined the trend to admit fewer and fewer patients to hospitals and to discharge patients more rapidly, limiting the length of patient terms in-house. Statistics show the amount of inpatient hospital care for the mentally ill decreased during the latter half of the twentieth century while the volume of mental health care needs increased. By 1994, only 26% of mental health care episodes were in 24-hour hospitals, down from 77% in 1955. This trend was consistent in various states and regions. Many analysts attribute the decreased need for hospital care to the approval and use of new psychiatric medicines. Deinstitutionalization itself represents a trend to more humane and liberal

Conclusion

treatment of mental health patients in community-based settings. It also represents a change from longer, custodial care to more expedient, outpatient care. The entire process is also associated with the societal problems of homelessness. Between 30-50% of homeless people in the United States are afflicted with mental illness. Life outside the institution after even a brief internment can be difficult for many, but deinstitutionalization was thought to lead to regaining freedom and making responsible choices for the future, helping patients become contributing and productive citizens. (104)

* * *

Changes started slowly then gained momentum as they reflected the philosophies of the Civil Rights Movement. During the 1960s, the average length of stay in mental institutions decreased by more than half. Community care facilities became more popular than long-term care institutions. Public opinion of mental illness changed for the better, but it was still stigmatized. Support groups have actively worked to reduce discrimination beginning as protest movements in the 1970s, with many of the participant's being ex-patients of mental institutions. They objected to involuntary commitment, the use of electroconvulsive therapy, antipsychotic medication, and coercive psychiatry. In 1996, President Clinton signed the Mental Health Parity Act, which endorsed NAMI's goal of equal insurance coverage and as hospitalization costs increased, both federal and state governments were motivated to find less expensive alternates to hospitalization.

It wasn't a perfect solution because nothing ever is but it was better than the past. Many psychiatric abuses continued to surface and community services were often fragmented; persons with distressed mental conditions were still put into prisons or became homeless, distrustful and resisted help. In the United States today, there are an estimated 7,467 mental support groups, self-help organizations and consumer operated services. The present status of the movement seems to indicate a preference for the term "survivor" with more than 60% of ex-patient groups reporting as supporting anti-psychiatry beliefs and who consider themselves psychiatric "survivors." Deinstitutionalizing continues today because the preference is now for the smaller community facility, and for greater freedom and personal responsibility. (105)

Miss X

She is long gone from this world now, but her 73 years of hospitalization certainly deserves our attention and even wonder. Maybe in an odd way Miss X had the last laugh as twelve of the fourteen institutions we explored shuttered their doors before she died. In effect, she outlasted them.

No record exists for the death of the patient simply known as Miss X, but it is likely her remains now reside in one of the thousands of unmarked graves in the long forgotten cemetery, of a mad-house. (106)

Thoughts of a Patient

Phebe B. Davis, spent over two years as a patient in The New York State Lunatic Asylum, at Utica. After her release she published a pamphlet to inform the public about the terrible abuses that she had endured while in "the house." At the end of her book was this poem-

Thoughts of a Patient
Suggested by hearing Dr. C. say, "You'll soon be well again."

"When shall it be?
In spring, when sleeping flowers awake,
And streams their icy fetters break,
And zephyrs gay unfold their wings,
And vernal sweetness 'round earth clings;
When natures tones I loved so well,
Then - then will I be well?"

"When shall it be?
It is when 'round my parents' hearth
Are mingled former tones of mirth?
And when no voice of grief is heard,
Nor is a sound of sadness stirred,
Save one short word, in sorrow tells,

An absent one remembered well:
Then - then shall I be well?"

"When shall it be?
When sunny hopes no more sustain
An aged mother's tottering frame,
And reasons fled her active brain,
And grief a manly brother slain;
When death has moved my sister home;
When all I loved, but self, are gone:
Then - then will I be well?"

"I shall be well!
I know - when earth has loosed her claims,
And naught that animates remains,
And the soul, that God to earth has lent,
Backward to Heaven its course hath bent -
And when around my new-made tomb
Is breathed affection's Farwell moan -
Yes! - Then I shall be well!"

Notes

(1) The History of Mental Illness, www. studentpulse.com

(2) IBID

(3) IBID

(4) Hippocrates www.Ancient History.about.com

(5) Foreign Afflictions www.Scientific American.com

(6) The Discovery of the Asylum Rothman, D., the Discovery of the Asylum. Boston: Little, Brown, 1971.

(7) Royal Bethlem Hospital www. Bethlem Heritage.org

(8) www.sciencemuseum.org/uk/philipepinel

(9) "The History of the York Retreat" www.The History of York.org

(10) "Moral Treatment" www.Sanctuaryweb.com

(11) Ordway, Janet Eddy. (1998).Dorothea Lynde Dix: A Woman Ahead of Her Time. Psychiatric News. Available online at:http://www.psych.org/

pnews/98-10-16/hx.html

(12) Kirkbride TS: Proceedings of the Third Meeting of the Association of Medical Superintendents of American Institutions for The Insane, Article V. New York, July 1848, p 91

(13) "Kirkbride Plan."2012. 4 Nov 2012. <http://en.wikipedia.org/wiki/ Kirkbride_Plan

(14) "Thomas Story Kirkbride"   www.alleghenylunaticasylum.com

(15) Tomes, Nancy A., "A Generous Confidence: Thomas Story Kirkbride and the Art of Asylum Keeping, 1840-1883. Cambridge University Press, 1984

(16)www.alleghanylunaticasylum.com/thomasstorykirkbride

(17)"Bellevue" www.history-magazine.comNew York: Harper and Brothers, 1882.

(18) New York Times, November 16, 1884.gov

(19) www.wikipedia.org/Bellevue/Hospital Center

(20) www.nyc.gov/Bellevue

(21) History of Roosevelt Island By Daniel Morales, www.eastriverhistory. web

(22) IBID

(23)"Blackwell's Island Lunatic Asylum." Harper's New Monthly Magazine Feb. 1866. Nyc10044.com. 4 Oct. 2011.

(24) Bly, Nellie. Ten Days in a Mad-House. New York: Ian L. Munro, 1887.

(25) Boardman, M.D., Samantha, and George J. Makari, M.D. "The Lunatic Asylum on Blackwell's Island and the New York Press."

Notes

(26)"Records Of the Monroe County Insane Asylum (1857-1891)."University of Rochester

(27)Medical Center Library. Web. 8 Nov 2012. <http://www.urmc. rochester.edu/hslt/miner/historical_services/archives/RecordGroups/ MonroeCountyInsaneAsylum.cfm>.

(28)"Rochester State Hospital."8 Nov 2012. http://www.opacity.us/site119_ rochester_state_hospital.htm>.

(29)The Remember Garden.8 Nov 2012. <http://www. memorialofrecovereddignity.org/documents/The_Remember_Garden.pdf>.

(30)"Poor Houses" Inmates of Willard Files blog, July 2012, Monroe County

(31) The Rolling Hills Asylum Official Website/VP web.com

(32) Rolling Hills, Bethany, New York Investigations by Long Island Paranormal Investigators: Rolling Hills, Bethany, New York

(33)"Cattaraugus Poor House Story" www.HistoricalGazette.com

(34) "Social Welfare History, Caring for paupers in 1881"www. socialwelfarehistory.org

(35)"The Stone House Asylum" www.Cattco.org/book

(36)"The Stone House Asylum" Reprinted with permission of Tom Woodman, Editor of the Daily Gazette genealogy.rootsweb.ancestry. com/~clifflamere/Cem/CEM-AlbAlmshouse.htm

(37) www.correctionshistory.org/Charles Clarke

(38) "The Stone House Asylum", Woodman/Daily Gazette

(39)The History of Albany Poorhouses http://www.poorhousestory.com/ALBANY.htm

(40)David Wagner, "Poor Relief and the Almshouse,"

(41)Luther, Roger. "Utica State Hospital". Web. 4 Nov 2012. <http://nysasylum.com/utica/index.htm>.

(42)"Amariah Brigham.". Web. 4 Nov 2012. <http://en.wikipedia.org/wiki/Amariah_Brigham>.

(43) Utica Psychiatric Institute.". Web. 4 Nov 2012. <http://en.wikipedia.org/wiki/Utica_Psychiatric_Center>

(44)"The Opal". Google Books. Web. 4 Nov 2012. <http://books.google.com/books/about/The_Opal.html?id=bMARAAAAYAAJ>.

(45)McKivigan, John. "The "Black Dream" of Gerrit Smith, New York Abolitionist .Nov 2012. <http://www.nyhistory.com/gerritsmith/dream.htm>.

(46) Artifact of the Month: "The Utica Crib". Western Illinois Museum, Web. 4 Nov 2012. <http://www.westernillinoismuseum.org/artifact_month/2011

(47)"The Old Main." 29 2010. Web. 4 Nov 2012. <http://newyorktraveler.net/the-main-or-utica-lunatic-asylum-ny/>.

(48) Disability History Museum, http://www.disabilitymuseum.org/dhm/edu/essay.html?id=60 (accessed date).

(49)James Thornton Correspondence Inclusive Dates: 1855-1866 Letters concerning James (Jimmy) Thornton of Cincinnatus, New York, a pupil at the New York Asylum for Idiots in Syracuse, from Dr. Hervey Wilbur and other staff at the institution to the boy's mother, Mary Thornton (later Mary Wheat).
Repository: Special Collections Research Center, Syracuse University Library
222 Waverly Avenues
Syracuse, NY 13244-2010
http://scrc.syr.edu

Notes

(50) IBID

(51)New York State Inebriate Asylum www.nysasylum.com

(52) IBID

(53)Binghamton State Hospital www.rootsweb.ancestry.com

(54) www.nysassylum.com/wet packing

(55)Binghamton Inebriate Asylum www.paranormalghostsociety.org

(56)"Echoes of Willard", Mary Rote

(57)The Inmates of Willard 1870 to 1900: A Genealogy Resource [Paperback] Linda S. Stuhler (Author) self published

(58) IBID http://www.echoesofwillard.com/willard-psychiatric-centre/

(59) "Our State Institutions" The New York Times, March 21, 1872

(60) "Inmates of Willard 1870-1900" http://inmatesofwillard.files.wordpress.com/2011/10/1916-willard-state-hospital.pdf

(61) IBID

(62) IBID Inmates of Willard 1870-1900 www.willardcemeterymemorialproject.com

(63) "The Female Hunter of Delaware County" Diane Anderson-Minshaw, Aug. 2, 2012 www.advocate.com

(64) "Hudson River State Hospital" http://www.forbidden-places.net

(65) "Health Affairs", 11, no.3 (1992):7-22, Gerald Grob

(66) IBID

(67) IBID

(68) "Hudson River State Hospital" www.asylumprojects.org

(69)www.crimezzz.net/serialkillers.com

(70) "The Asylums"! The Insane Foundations of Columbia University.", Bowery Boys. Web. 27 Dec 2012. <http://theboweryboys.blogspot. com/2009/05/insane-foundations-of-columbia.html>.

(71)"Dr. Thomas Story Kirkbride" Proceedings of the Third Meeting of the Association of Medical Superintendents of American Institutions for The Insane, Article V. New York, July 1848, p 91

(72) "Buffalo State Hospital" http://nysasylum.com/bpc/bpchist.htm

(73) "Reports of Abuse at Buffalo Insane Asylum March 3, 1881 the New York Times

(74) "Haunted Buffalo State Hospital" www.opacity.us/image2151_dark_ asylum.htm

(75) "Halloween at Murder Creek" http://artvoice.com Buck Quigley

(76) "History of Middletown Homeopathic Hospital http://history.tomrue.net

(77) "Homeopathic Healing" http://en.wikipedia.org/wiki/Homeopathy

(78) "History of Middletown Homeopathic Hospital" http://en.wikapedia.org

(79) IBID

(80) IBID

(81) "History of Middletown Homeopathic Hospital"

(82)"The History of Matteawan State Hospital for the Criminally Insane" www.hudsonvalleyruins.org

(83) Ordway, Janet Eddy. (1998).Dorothea Lynde Dix: A Woman Ahead of Her Time. Psychiatric News. Available online at:http://www.psych.org/pnews/98-10-16/hx.html

(84) Nellie Bly:"Charles Dickens visit to Blackwell Island Asylum 1842" Bly, Nellie: Ten Days in a Mad House, New York Ian L. Munro 1887

(85) "Inside The Auburn Prison" Cayuga County Historical Society www.co.cayuga.ny.us

(86) IBID

(87) "The History of Matteawan Hospital www.hudsonvalleyruins.org

(88) IBID

(89) "The Trial of Harry Thaw", Mackenzie, F.A., Geoffrey Bles

(90) Serial Killer Lizzie Halliday, "The Worst Woman on Earth The Unknown History of Misandry" http://unknownmisandry.blogspot.com

(91) "On this day in NY history: Bloomingdale Lunatic Asylum opened, future site of Columbia University." . N.p.. Web. 27 Dec 2012. <http://www.examiner.com/article/on-this-day-ny-history-bloomingdale-lunatic-asylum-opened-future-site-of-columbia-university>.

(92) "Bloomingdale Insane Asylum." . N.p.. Web. 27 Dec 2012. <http://en.wikipedia.org/wiki/Bloomingdale_Insane_Asylum>.

(93) "Julius Chambers." . N.p.. Web. 27 Dec 2012. <http://en.wikipedia.org/wiki/Julius_Chambers>.

(94)"Undercover Reporting." . N.p.. Web. 27 Dec 2012. <http://dlib.nyu.edu/undercover/bloomingdale-asylum-exposé-julius-chambers-new-york-tribune>.

(95)"Charles Deas." . N.p.. Web. 27 Dec 2012. <http://en.wikipedia.org/wiki/Charles_Deas>.

(96)"Western Pioneer." . Westword. Web. 27 Dec 2012. <http://www.westword.com/2010-08-19/calendar/western-pioneer/>.

(97) www.asylumprojects.org/Topeka_State

(98) IBID

(99) www.actionforaccess.mohistory.org

(100) www.cracked.com

(101)www.archives.nysed.gov

(102) www.uvm.edu/eugenics

(103) www.ncbi.nlm.nih.gov/world psychiatry

(104)www.ssa.gov/policy/docs/medicaire

(105) www.wps.prenhall.com/wps/media/objects

(106) asylums project/Topeka State

Bibliography

Books

Andrews, Jonathan "The History of Bethlem", London, Routledge, 1997

Bly, Nellie "Ten Days in a Madhouse, Feigning Insanity in Order to Reveal Asylum Horrors", New York, Norman Munro, 1887

Bynum, W.F. The Anatomy of Madness", Essays in the History of Psychiatry, W.F. Bynum, Tavistock Publications, London & New York, 1985
Chesler, Phyllis, "Women and Madness", New York: Doubleday, 1972.

Dwyer, Ellen "Homes for the mad: life inside two nineteenth-century asylums
Rutgers University Press, 1987

Geller, Jeffrey L. and Harris, Maxine "Women of the Asylum", New York: Anchor Books, 1994.

Grob, Gerald, "The Mad Among Us: A History of the Care of America's Mentally Ill, New York, Free Press, 1994

Jackson, Kenneth T, The Encyclopedia of New York, Yale University Press, New Haven and London, 1995

Johnson-Braden, Ann "Out of Bedlam", the Truth about Deinstitutionalization, Basic Books, 1990

Reiss, Benjamin, "Theaters of Madness: Insane Asylums and Nineteenth-Century American Culture "University of Chicago Press, 2008

Rothman, David "The Discovery of the Asylum: Social Order and Disorder
in the New Republic, Boston, Little Brown 1971

Scull, A "Madhouse a Tragic Tale of Megalomania and Modern Medicine.
New Haven and London: Yale University Press, 2005.

Shorter, Edward "A History of Psychiatry from the Era of the Asylum to the
Age of Prozac", New York: Wiley, 1997

Szaza, Thomas S. "The Age of Madness":The History of Involuntary Mental
Hospitalization, London, Routledge and Keegan 1975

Wagner, D., "The Poorhouse": America's Forgotten Institution, Rowan-Lit-
tlefield, Latham MD2005.
Yanni, Carla, "The Architecture of Madness: Insane Asylums in the United
States"
U of Minnesota Press, 2007

Journals and Magazines

"Reform and Curability in American Insane Asylums of the 1800's", Alison
R. Brown, Volume 11/Issue 1, 2010

"The Inmates of Willard", 1870-1900, A Genealogy Resource, Dec. 20, 2011-
A Blog

"The Female Hunter of Delaware County",Diane Anderson, Aug 2, 2012
www.advocate.com

"A Visit to the Lunatic Asylum on Blackwell Island". Harper's Magazine
Weekly, March 19, 1858

Bibliography

"Almshouses and Insane Asylums of Hudson and Columbia County", Columbia County Historical Society

"Abandoned Suitcases", Hunter Oatman, November 5, 2012, Stanford Collectors Weekly

"Nellie Bly, Dare Devil Reporter", Sean McCollum, March 2012, Scholastic. com

"Two Years and Three Months in the New York State Lunatic Asylum at Utica": Phoebe Davis, the Evening Chronicle Book and Job Office, Delaine Buildings, 93 Pages, 1855
"Witching Hour, New York City Lunatic Asylum", Jade Wick, October 5, 2011

"The Lunatic Asylum on Blackwell Island", Samantha Boardman, American Journal of Psychiatry, 2007

"Records of the Monroe County Insane Asylum, (1857-1891)" University of Rochester Medical Center, Christopher Hoolihan, 2012

"The Most Famous and Notorious Insane Asylums in History", Jeremy Taylor, Feb. 2, 2010, Huff Post Weird News

"Hudson Valley Psychiatric Hospitals and Insane Asylums", C.J. Hughes, Sept. 13, 2011 Hudson Valley Magazine

"Rochester History", published quarterly by Rochester Public Library.

"Rochester's Early Hospitals", Rochester General Health System, Bob Dickson

"Rochester's History", An Illustrated Timeline

Blogs &Internet

Ancestry.com

Advocate.com

HudsonValleyRuins.com

Inmatesofwillard.com

Wikipedia.com

Correctional History.org

Scholastic.com

Paranormal Investigations

"Rolling Hills Asylum, Investigation by Long Island" Paranormal Investigators, Aug 2007

"Haunted Binghamton Inebriate Asylum", Amy Brown Dec 12, 2010

About the Author

Michael Keene worked for twenty-five years in the financial services industry as a financial advisor. He is the author of "Folklore and Legends of Rochester, The Mystery of Hoodoo Corner" and "Murder, Mayhem and Madness, 150 Years of Crime and Punishment in Western New York." He is also the producer of the award-winning documentary series, "Visions, True Stories of Spiritualism, Secret Societies & Murder". He lives in Pittsford, New York with his wife Diana and their daughter Michele, and grandson, Joshua. His website address is http://www.ad-hoc-productions.com and email is: info@ad-hoc-visions.com

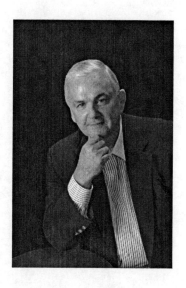

CPSIA information can be obtained at www.ICGtesting.com
Printed in the USA
BVOW02s2241120314

347467BV00006B/97/P